MEDICAL
EXAMINATION REVIEW

NEUROLOGY

TENTH EDITION

D1528022

MEDICAL EXAMINATION REVIEW

NEUROLOGY

TENTH EDITION

Paul S. Slosberg, MD
Associate Clinical Professor of Neurology
Mount Sinai School of Medicine
New York

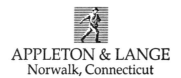

APPLETON & LANGE
Norwalk, Connecticut

ISBN 0 8385 5778 3

93 94 95 96 97 / 10 9 8 7 6 5 4 3 2

Prentice Hall International (UK) Limited, *London*
Prentice Hall of Australia Pty. Limited, *Sydney*
Prentice Hall Canada, Inc., *Toronto*
Prentice Hall Hispanoamericana, S.A., *Mexico*
Prentice Hall of India Private Limited, *New Delhi*
Prentice Hall of Japan, Inc., *Tokyo*
Simon & Schuster Asia Pte. Ltd., *Singapore*
Editora Prentice Hall do Brasil Ltda., *Rio de Janeiro*
Prentice Hall, *Englewood Cliffs, New Jersey*

Library of Congress Cataloging-in-Publication Data

Slosberg, Paul S.
  Medical examination review of neurology / Paul S. Slosberg. —
10th ed.
    p.   cm.
  Rev. ed of: Neurology. 9th ed. c1988.
  Includes bibliographical references.
  ISBN 0–8385–5778–3
    1. Neurology—Examinations, questions, etc. I. Slosberg, Paul
S.,   Neurology. II. Title.
    [DNLM: 1. Neurology—examination questions.   WL 18 S888m 1993]
  RC356.S56   1993
  616.8′076—dc20
  DNLM/DLC
  for Library of Congress   93–10813
                                                                  CIP

Acquisitions Editor: Jamie L. Mount
Production Editor: Sondra Greenfield
Designer: Kathy Hornyak

Contents

Preface

This tenth edition of *Neurology* has been substantially revised and updated to keep in step with current trends in medical education and the continuing expansion of scientific knowledge. It is designed to help you prepare for course examinations, such as the United States Medical Licensing Examination Step 2, the Federation Licensing Examination (FLEX), the Foreign Medical Graduate Examination in the Medical Sciences (FMGEMS), and other objective exams.

The range of subjects included in this volume is based on the content outline of the National Board of Medical Examiners, which develops the question pool for the tests mentioned above, and reflects the scope and depth of what is taught in medical schools today. The questions themselves are organized in broad categories to give you a representative sampling of the material covered in course work, while helping you define those general areas to which you need to devote attention. For your convenience in selective study, the answers (with commentary and references) follow each section of questions.

Each question has been scrutinized by specialists to verify that it is relevant and current. The author's care in item construction gives you questions that will provide good practice in familiarizing yourself with the format of objective-type tests. Questions of each type—one best response, matching, multiple true-false, and so on—are grouped together. They are modeled as closely as possible after those used on the United States Medical Licensing Examination Step 2.

Using this book, you may identify areas of strength and weakness in your own command of the subject. Specific references to widely used textbooks allow you to return to the authoritative source for further study. This volume supplements the lettered answers with brief explanations intended to prompt you to think about the choices, correct and incorrect, to put the answers in broadened perspective, and to add to your fund of knowledge. A complete bibliography appears at the end of the book. The questions and answers, taken together, emphasize problem solving and application of underlying principles as well as retention of factual knowledge.

1

Vascular Disease

DIRECTIONS (Questions 1–56): Each of the questions or incomplete statements below is followed by five suggested answers or completions. Select the ONE lettered answer or completion that is BEST in each case.

1. Patients with subarachnoid hemorrhage and negative angiograms
    A. have a poor prognosis
    B. have a prognosis similar to that of ruptured aneurysm
    C. have a prognosis similar to that of ruptured arteriovenous malformation
    D. have a good prognosis
    E. will probably be found eventually to harbor a brain tumor

2. Arteriovenous malformations
    A. coexist with intracranial aneurysms in approximately 20% to 30% of cases
    B. may enlarge markedly without clinical worsening
    C. rarely present without subarachnoid hemorrhage
    D. are visualized well on angiography, poorly on CT scan
    E. none of the above

3. The patient suddenly feels dizzy, vomits, and has difficulty swallowing. On examination, he has a Horner's syndrome plus analgesia and thermoanesthesia on one side of the face, with similar sensory deficits on the opposite side of the body. He most likely has suffered
 A. thrombosis of the anterior cerebral artery or middle cerebral artery
 B. thrombosis of the posterior inferior cerebellar artery or vertebral artery
 C. hemorrhage into the internal capsule
 D. embolism of the posterior cerebral artery
 E. occlusion of one carotid artery

4. Acute paralysis of the left lower extremity with lesser involvement of the left upper extremity would be most likely to occur in
 A. anterior cerebral artery occlusion
 B. middle cerebral artery occlusion
 C. posterior cerebral artery occlusion
 D. posterior inferior cerebellar artery occlusion
 E. anterior spinal artery occlusion

5. Ipsilateral transient amblyopia with contralateral hemimotor and hemisensory defects occurs most often in
 A. internal carotid artery disease
 B. vertebrobasilar artery disease
 C. middle cerebral artery disease
 D. posterior choroidal artery disease
 E. A and C but not B

6. The most common cause of nontraumatic bleeding into the subarachnoid space is
 A. aneurysm
 B. arteriovenous malformation
 C. intracranial tumors
 D. blood dyscrasias
 E. none of the above

7. A major factor in the origin of cerebral aneurysm is
 A. trauma
 B. congenital-developmental weakness
 C. syphilis

    D. septic emboli
    E. none of the above

8. In the adult, most intracranial aneurysms occur at the
    A. anterior communicating and internal carotid arteries
    B. vertebrobasilar and internal carotid arteries
    C. middle cerebral and vertebrobasilar arteries
    D. pericallosal arteries
    E. none of the above

9. Arteriovenous malformation of the vein of Galen
    A. is treated surgically with almost uniformly excellent results
    B. may rarely be accompanied by cardiac failure
    C. after operation is rarely complicated by subdural hematoma
    D. is seldom congenital
    E. none of the above

10. The most common syndrome in lacunar stroke is
    A. dysarthria-clumsy hand
    B. pure motor hemiplegia
    C. pure hemianopsia
    D. ipsilateral ataxia and hemiparesis
    E. pure aphasia

11. In adults, cerebral embolism is commonly caused by
    A. heart disease
    B. air emboli
    C. neoplastic thrombi
    D. fat emboli secondary to fracture
    E. septic pulmonary disease

12. Occlusion of the internal carotid artery
    A. usually produces nystagmus
    B. may cause no symptoms
    C. may cause a Brown-Séquard syndrome
    D. may cause no symptoms unless the contralateral carotid artery is also occluded, at which time symptoms are inevitable
    E. does not produce coma initially

13. In cases of occlusion of the internal carotid artery
   A. one may hear a bruit in the neck in internal carotid but not external carotid disease
   B. hypersensitive carotid sinus reflex is almost always absent
   C. transient ipsilateral amblyopia often occurs; homonymous hemianopsia occurs in about half the cases
   D. transient ischemic attacks last less than 24 hours
   E. ophthalmodynamometry is abnormal as often as it is in vertebrobasilar disease

14. Association of cardiac dysfunction in cerebrovascular disease is
   A. rare
   B. unknown
   C. occasional
   D. frequent
   E. one-to-one relationship

15. The syndrome of anterior spinal artery thrombosis
   A. occurs in Hodgkin's disease
   B. includes paralysis and dissociated sensory loss
   C. is usually due to lues or tuberculosis
   D. A and B but not C
   E. A and C but not B

16. Ruptured intracranial aneurysm does not present frequently with
   A. severe headache
   B. nausea and vomiting
   C. loss of consciousness
   D. nuchal rigidity
   E. none of the above

17. In patients with known intracranial aneurysm, the incidence of multiple aneurysm is generally felt to be
   A. 10% to 25%
   B. negligible
   C. 50% to 60%
   D. 2% to 25%
   E. none of the above

18. In the management of subarachnoid hemorrhage with angiographically proven aneurysm
   - **A.** medical treatment with hypotension is very effective
   - **B.** surgical treatment with carotid ligation has been discarded
   - **C.** surgical treatment with clipping, ligating, trapping, packing, wrapping, wiring, magnifying loops, and dissecting microscopes has been proven effective for most cases treated within 24 to 48 hours of the bleed
   - **D.** surgical treatments with pilojection, plastic encasement, proximal occlusion, electrical thrombosis, balloon thrombosis, magnetic thrombosis, body-cooling apparatus, and hyperbaric chambers are all widely used
   - **E.** antifibrinolytic drugs are used to prevent normal pressure hydrocephalus

19. With regard to long-term prognosis, fatal recurrence in subarachnoid hemorrhage due to aneurysm
   - **A.** is very unlikely with long-term medical-hypotensive therapy
   - **B.** does not occur with macrosurgical therapy
   - **C.** does not occur with microsurgical therapy
   - **D.** is least likely with carotid ligation
   - **E.** is least likely with the Selverstone clamp

20. In the treatment of subarachnoid hemorrhage due to aneurysm
   - **A.** the International Randomized Study (1972) reported that medical treatment with hypotension was the best treatment
   - **B.** microneurosurgical methods, hyperbaric chambers, and body cooling have eliminated the problem of the post-operative "vegetable" result
   - **C.** a 61-year-old hypertensive, lethargic patient with spasm would be accepted by most surgeons as a good risk, especially for early surgery
   - **D.** use of the dissecting microscope is endorsed by all leading aneurysm surgeons
   - **E.** patients who do not have an operation face, as a group, an annual mortality due to recurrent hemorrhage

21. Atherosclerosis in the arteries to the brain
    A. is usually evident in the third decade of life
    B. includes intimal lipid deposition without fibrous tissue over-growth
    C. frequently involves the region about 1 cm below the common carotid bifurcation
    D. infrequently involves the origin of the middle cerebral artery
    E. infrequently involves the vertebral arteries just after they enter the skull

22. Besides cerebral atherosclerosis
    A. anomalies of the circle of Willis, especially involving the posterior communicating arteries, occur in about one-fifth of the population and must be considered
    B. collagen-vascular disease is the second most frequent vascular inflammation producing cerebral infarction
    C. Takayasu's disease involves the origin of the cerebral arteries from the aortic arch and its branches
    D. frequently acute bacterial pharyngeal infections lead to carotid vasculitis and cerebral infarction
    E. Takayasu's disease is improved significantly in most cases through the use of either steroids or anticonvulsants

23. Infarction by cerebral embolus
    A. in a 66-year-old man would most commonly be caused by rheumatic heart disease with mitral stenosis and atrial fibrillation
    B. is commonly caused by fat, myocardial infarction with mural thrombi, and atrial fibrillation of unknown cause
    C. occurs in subacute bacterial endocarditis, thyrotoxicosis with atrial fibrillation, and nonbacterial thrombotic endocarditis
    D. frequently involves a patent foramen ovale
    E. is less often hemorrhagic than is infarction due to atherosclerotic occlusion

24. Cerebral emboli
    A. can produce brain abscess, encephalitis, or mycotic aneurysm
    B. cause neuropathologic changes that are identical to the changes found in infarction from other causes

C. can cause transient ischemic attacks provided that some degree of vascular obstruction is already present
D. cause infarction even when minute vessels are occluded
E. are retrievable at autopsy in almost all cases

25. Cerebral venous thrombosis
    A. can cause infarction if a major venous sinus is involved
    B. does not cause infarction if only cortical veins are involved
    C. of surface vessels is usually not associated with cerebral or subdural abscess
    D. is not associated with head injury or dehydration
    E. is not associated with polycythemia vera or leukemia

26. Cerebral venous thrombosis
    A. of the cavernous sinus is invariably unilateral
    B. is most commonly caused by infection of the mastoid, frontal sinus, or subdural space
    C. of the superior sagittal sinus anteriorly produces marked congestion of both cerebral hemispheres, limited to the cortex
    D. of the cavernous sinus is not followed by meningitis
    E. does not occur in the puerperium

27. In evaluating the role of hypertension in cerebral infarction, a rapid rise in blood pressure
    A. in animals causes constriction of small cerebral vessels but no infarction
    B. in humans has not been proved to be distinctly involved in the production of cerebral infarction
    C. causes an increase in cerebrovascular resistance, and in model experiments even this, plus stenosis, does not reduce blood flow significantly
    D. is probably the single biggest risk factor in stroke
    E. none of the above

28. In the diagnosis of cerebral embolism
- **A.** abrupt onset of paretic symptoms is often preceded by headache
- **B.** normal CSF protein without cells suggests the possibility of subacute bacterial endocarditis
- **C.** normal sinus rhythm tends to exclude the diagnosis
- **D.** convulsions commonly occur at the onset
- **E.** prolonged loss of consciousness usually occurs

29. In cerebral venous thrombosis
- **A.** paresis and hemisensory loss are uncommon
- **B.** postpartum cerebral infarction is likely present
- **C.** headache and delirium are common; diplopia and convulsions are rare
- **D.** fever would not be expected
- **E.** papilledema is uncommon

30. In cerebral venous thrombosis
- **A.** superior sagittal sinus occlusion has been followed by pseudotumor cerebri
- **B.** cavernous sinus occlusion typically presents with proptosis and orbital chemosis, but eye pain is uncommon
- **C.** lateral sinus involvement, which is still common, presents with mastoid tenderness, dysphagia, dysphonia, and weakness of the sternomastoid and trapezius muscles
- **D.** below the age of 10, fewer infarctions are found than are found in arterial occlusion
- **E.** headache and leukocytosis are unlikely

31. In the patient with cerebral infarction
- **A.** myocardial infarction, hypertension, or diabetes mellitus is often found
- **B.** peripheral vascular disease is found in almost half of the cases
- **C.** the diastolic pressure is above 100 mm Hg in three-fourths of the cases
- **D.** a previous cerebral episode has occurred in more than half the cases
- **E.** almost all antecedent strokes had taken place three to five years earlier

32. Lumbar puncture in a patient with cerebral infarction
- **A.** differentiates between intracranial hemorrhage and hemorrhagic infarction
- **B.** may show a protein elevation due to diabetes mellitus
- **C.** frequently shows CSF pressures in the 200- to 220-mm range
- **D.** may show a slightly lower protein level in basilar artery disease
- **E.** may show a protein elevation of 200 mg/100 mL if the infarction is massive

33. In the patient with brain infarction
- **A.** CT or MRI scans have replaced pneumoencephalography in radiographic diagnosis
- **B.** CT or MRI scans have not replaced EEG in diagnosis
- **C.** CT or MRI scans have not replaced echoencephalography in diagnosis
- **D.** CT scan differentiates normal from infarcted brain during the first few days
- **E.** on average, CT scan will accurately detect lesions 2 mm in diameter or larger in 90% of cases

34. In the course of cerebral infarction
- **A.** cerebral edema complicates the situation in about three-fourths of the cases
- **B.** decrease in awareness may be due to edema, fever, sedatives, or electrolyte imbalance
- **C.** recovery from impaired neurologic function may continue for as long as several months
- **D.** malnutrition has no significant effect
- **E.** tranquilizers have no appreciable effect

35. In the prognosis of cerebral infarction
- **A.** age but not degree of neurologic disability is an important determinant of initial mortality
- **B.** once the stroke has happened, hypertension and diabetes do not alter the outlook
- **C.** a very important limiting factor in survival is the degree of cardiovascular disease
- **D.** approximately one-half die with their first attack
- **E.** about half of the patients who survive atherosclerotic infarction have a second attack within the next one to seven years

36. Anticoagulation
    A.   must be discontinued even when minor bleeding occurs
    B.   usually does not provoke bleeding unless the prothrombin time has become four to five times the control value
    C.   is best begun initially with a coumarin anticoagulant alone
    D.   causes serious hemorrhagic complications in 15% to 20% of cases
    E.   has a mortality rate of 8% to 10%

37. In hypertensive encephalopathy
    A.   the outlook has not been significantly altered by the use of hypotensive therapy
    B.   urea nitrogen usually is in excess of 100 mg%
    C.   edema, small infarctions, petechial hemorrhages, and massive hemorrhages are found at postmortem
    D.   papilledema is seldom present
    E.   the CSF is normal

38. In nontraumatic intracranial hemorrhage, one does not find
    A.   bleeding, which may begin at a subarachnoid surface vessel and penetrate the brain secondarily
    B.   bleeding, which may begin in brain tissue and extend into the subarachnoid space or ventricular system
    C.   berry aneurysms, which occur at the anterior portion of the circle of Willis
    D.   berry aneurysms, which occur relatively rarely in infants
    E.   none of the above

39. Berry aneurysms
    A.   enlarge with time, presumably under the stress of arterial blood pressure
    B.   are not more frequent in patients who are hypertensive
    C.   have been shown to rupture as a result of atheromatous plaques in their walls plus the presence of clots lining them
    D.   occur in multiple fashion in 1 out of every 10 patients who harbor aneurysms
    E.   frequently reach 4 to 5 cm in diameter

40. Fusiform aneurysms
    A.   occur more often along the carotid artery than along the basilar artery

    B. often compress cranial nerves
    C. frequently hemorrhage and are often fatal
    D. do not compress the brain itself
    E. are not due to atherosclerosis

41. Mycotic aneurysms
    A. occur at the site of local necrotic vasculitis where an embolus had lodged
    B. tend to be single
    C. are the only aneurysms found proximally in the larger branches of the middle cerebral artery
    D. do not bleed
    E. are produced by nonseptic emboli

42. Arteriovenous malformations
    A. are usually supplied by one parent cerebral artery
    B. may cover most of one cerebral hemisphere or occupy an entire cerebellar lobe
    C. are on the surface of the brain and therefore cause subarachnoid hemorrhage but not intracerebral hemorrhage
    D. do not expand unless hemorrhage has occurred
    E. frequently cause bleeding in the brain stem

43. In intracranial hemorrhage due to hypertensive vascular disease
    A. thickening, and especially fibrinoid degeneration of arterioles, may be significant
    B. the location is most often cerebellar and cerebral; least often brain stem
    C. brain stem lesions involve vertebrobasilar circumferential vessels more often than paramedian perforated vessels
    D. the location is most often the brain stem and cerebellum
    E. fibrinoid degeneration is probably least important

44. Hemorrhage in brain tumors occurs
    A. in either primary or metastatic lesions
    B. most often in slow-growing tumors with much vascular overgrowth
    C. most often in slow-growing tumors and hypernephroma
    D. least often in metastatic lung tumors
    E. least often in pituitary adenomas (among the more benign neoplasms)

45. In subarachnoid hemorrhage, the released blood does not
- **A.** cause meningeal exudation, scarring, impaired CSF absorption, and eventual communicating hydrocephalus
- **B.** irritate blood vessels, meninges, and brain
- **C.** produce cardiac arrhythmia via descending autonomic discharges
- **D.** cause hypertension via descending autonomic discharges
- **E.** none of the above

46. In subarachnoid hemorrhage, ischemia and infarction occur
- **A.** but are readily prevented by medications
- **B.** and are found least often in the region of the brain supplied by the artery with the ruptured aneurysm
- **C.** and have been attributed to spasm secondary to irritation by the released blood plus vessel injury; also, surgical manipulation may cause severe spasm
- **D.** but do not result in a postoperative vegetable-like existence
- **E.** none of the above

47. Intracerebral hemorrhage
- **A.** is most often caused by arteriovenous malformation
- **B.** invariably damages much neural tissue in the area of bleeding
- **C.** is most often caused by hypertensive vascular disease or ruptured aneurysm
- **D.** does not always produce cerebral edema
- **E.** produces gradual brain enlargement leading to tentorial herniation

48. In subarachnoid hemorrhage
- **A.** convulsions may occur at the onset
- **B.** the most common localizing neurologic sign is a hypertonic hemiplegia or hemiparesis with a Babinski sign
- **C.** the most conspicuous sign is papilledema
- **D.** subhyaloid hemorrhages are almost always bilateral
- **E.** body temperature most often reaches 40°C but does not exceed it

49. Aneurysmal bleeding involving the
- **A.** middle cerebral artery tends to produce hemimotor and hemisensory defects

    B. posterior communicating artery tends to produce ptosis, diplopia, mydriasis, and impaired abduction
    C. anterior cerebral-anterior communicating artery area tends to produce bilateral extremity (especially upper) paresis
    D. cavernous portion of the carotid artery is common
    E. none of the above

50. In the diagnosis of bleeding due to ruptured arteriovenous malformation
    A. an antecedent history of focal seizures, focal neurologic signs, and unilateral headache is suggestive
    B. the clinical findings differ from those of ruptured aneurysm
    C. a bruit may be found with equal frequency in aneurysm and arteriovenous malformation
    D. seizures at the onset of bleeding are nearly always generalized
    E. bleeding into the surrounding brain is unusual

51. In the diagnosis of intracerebral hemorrhage
    A. the differentiation from hemorrhagic infarction can be made by lumbar puncture in almost every case
    B. the onset is usually gradual
    C. loss of consciousness soon after onset is frequent
    D. headache occurs as often as it does in cerebral infarction
    E. thalamic hemorrhage frequently causes downward gaze paralysis

52. Bleeding in the posterior fossa, at onset and
    A. if brain stem, may cause impaired consciousness, large pupils, and irregular respiration
    B. if cerebellar, may cause impaired consciousness, vertigo, large pupils, and irregular respiration
    C. if cerebellar, sometimes includes occipital headache, diplopia, nystagmus, and ataxia hours before loss of consciousness
    D. if brain stem, is usually at the medullary level
    E. if brain stem, loss of consciousness is often preceded by severe headache and diplopia

53. In a traumatic spinal tap, the CSF
  - **A.** when centrifuged, may have a pink supernatant due to the presence of oxyhemoglobin
  - **B.** when centrifuged, may have a yellow supernatant due to the presence of bilirubin
  - **C.** may show 10 white blood cells for every 1000 red blood cells
  - **D.** may be examined, for confirmation, by spectrophotometry
  - **E.** reacts negatively with benzidine

54. Arteriography in intracranial bleeding may demonstrate
  - **A.** an aneurysm of a distal branch of a middle or anterior cerebral artery, raising the possibility of mycotic aneurysm
  - **B.** irregularity in the outline of an aneurysm, the most reliable evidence of bleeding in cases of multiple aneurysm
  - **C.** delayed arterial filling and venous drainage in arteriovenous malformations
  - **D.** intracerebral hematomas in almost 100% of the cases
  - **E.** aneurysms in almost 100% of the cases

55. In the treatment of subarachnoid hemorrhage due to large, arteriovenous malformations that have not bled
  - **A.** medical management is the treatment of choice for most cases
  - **B.** carotid artery ligation or parent vessel ligation is the treatment of choice for most cases
  - **C.** amputation of the portion of the brain containing the anomaly is the treatment of choice in most cases
  - **D.** the chance for rebleeding is the same as that for aneurysm
  - **E.** bleeding carries a mortality comparable to that of aneurysm

56. In the treatment of intracerebral hemorrhage
  - **A.** surgical treatment is the treatment of choice
  - **B.** no matter what treatment is used, a large percentage of patients in deep, persistent coma do not survive
  - **C.** the results of surgical removal of an intracerebral hematoma caused by ruptured aneurysm are more encouraging than the results when bleeding is due to hypertensive vascular disease

D. the disorder can now be managed satisfactorily in most cases

E. patients in coma frequently survive

DIRECTIONS (Questions 57 through 61): Each group of questions below consists of lettered headings followed by a list of numbered words or statements. For each numbered word or statement, select the ONE lettered heading that is most closely associated with it. Each lettered heading may be selected once, more than once, or not at all.

A. Bilateral visual blurring
B. Diplopia
C. Ataxia
D. Vertigo
E. Bilateral, alternating, or "crossed" motor and sensory symptoms

---

57. Vestibular nuclei—medulla and pons

58. Cerebellum or cerebellar connections

59. Oculomotor nuclei—midbrain and pons

60. Long motor and sensory tracts, cranial nerve nuclei

61. Visual cortex—occipital lobe

Answers and Discussion

1. **(D)** The mortality has been found by some authors to be approximately one-tenth that of patients with hemorrhage and demonstrable aneurysm. Four-vessel angiography must have been performed and (infrequently) if there is a suspicion of primary spinal subarachnoid hemorrhage, the latter must be ruled out by appropriate studies. **(Ref. 5, p. 237)**

2. **(B)** Instead of presenting with subarachnoid hemorrhage, arteriovenous malformations may initially cause seizures, headache, etc., or may be found incidental to another lesion. It should be noted that at no age are arteriovenous malformations the most likely cause of hemorrhage. There is an occasional coexistence with intracranial aneurysms. MRI (angiography) can be helpful. **(Ref. 5, pp. 240–242)**

3. **(B)** Nystagmus is found along with ipsilateral incoordination and ipsilateral paralysis of the soft palate, pharynx, and vocal cord. This is probably more often due to thrombosis of one vertebral artery and is the lateral medullary (or Wallenberg's) syndrome. **(Ref. 4, p. 292)**

4. **(A)** The anterior cerebral artery supplies the paracentral lobule. Therefore, anterior cerebral artery obstruction may cause a contralateral lower limb monoplegia. Sometimes the contralateral upper limb is affected resulting in a grasp reflex. Posterior cerebral artery occlusion causes crossed homonymous hemianopsia. Middle cerebral artery occlusion causes motor, sensory, and speech

defects which are indistinguishable from those due to occlusion of the internal carotid artery. (**Ref.** 4, p. 291)

5. (A) A focal or generalized convulsive disorder may occur. This may be recurrent and transitory, a clinical picture described as "stuttering hemiplegia." However, the internal carotid artery may be completely occluded and yet cause no symptoms. Permanent blindness of the ipsilateral eye is rare. (**Ref.** 4, p. 290)

6. (A) The demonstration of a specific cause depends to a great extent on the thoroughness of angiography; ideally, all four major vessels should be visualized. Other uncommon causes of nontraumatic subarachnoid hemorrhage include infection (eg, bacterial or tuberculous meningitis, syphilis, herpes encephalitis), arterial or venous hemorrhagic infarction and vasculitis (eg, systemic lupus erythematosus, polyarteritis nodosa, Henoch-Schönlein syndrome). (**Ref.** 5, p. 242)

7. (B) Defects in media and elastica have been cited, along with a mechanical factor. The role of atherosclerosis is uncertain. Some workers report that aneurysms occur in up to 4% of routine adult autopsies. Hypertension contributes to the formation and rupture of aneurysms. (**Ref.** 5, p. 235)

8. (A) This is the case whether angiographic or postmortem data are used. Aneurysms of the posterior part of the circle of Willis occur most often at the apical bifurcation of the basilar artery. Some reports indicate a higher incidence of posterior Circle aneurysms in infants. (**Ref.** 5, p. 235)

9. (E) Symptoms and signs usually develop in infancy or early childhood. These occur when a branch of the carotid or vertebrobasilar arterial system communicates directly with this vein. Seizures and hydrocephalus occur especially in infancy; the older child or adult experiences a greater frequency of headache and subarachnoid hemorrhage. (**Ref.** 5, p. 242)

10. (B) These occlusions have been said to be the end result of long-standing hypertension. Pure motor hemiplegia, pure hemisensory stroke, and pseudobulbar palsy are all relatively more common than either ipsilateral ataxia with hemiparesis or dysarthria-clumsy hand syndrome. When the lacunar syndrome can be explained adequately by hypertensive disease, the only specific therapy indicated is hypertension control. (**Ref.** 5, p. 215)

11. **(A)** In adults, this is especially due to atrial fibrillation or myocardial infarction. In children, this is commonly associated with valvular heart disease (rheumatic or congenital) and superimposed endocarditis. Air embolism usually follows injuries or surgical procedures involving lungs, dural sinuses, or jugular veins. Fat embolism is rare and is almost always due to bone fracture. (**Ref.** 5, pp. 184–185)

12. **(B)** This may occur because of carotid-carotid and carotid-vertebrobasilar anastomoses. At the other extreme, massive cerebral infarction may occur. The adequacy or inadequacy of the collateral circulation presumably is a major factor. Nystagmus in central nervous system lesions indicates posterior fossa dysfunction. Brown-Séquard syndrome indicates cord hemisection. (**Ref.** 5, p. 211)

13. **(D)** The diagnostic value of a bruit has been debated. Several writers report that 4% of Americans older than 45 evince carotid bifurcation bruit. Reversible ischemic neurologic deficit (RIND) has been applied to symptoms that improve within 24 hours but leave some minor neurologic abnormality. (**Ref.** 5, pp. 192, 205–206)

14. **(D)** In addition, hypertension is extremely common in cerebral hemorrhage or infarction; the blood pressure is usually normal in embolism. In some patients with subarachnoid hemorrhage, cardiac conduction defects and dysrhythmias or pulmonary edema occur. (**Ref.** 5, p. 191)

15. **(D)** Hodgkin's disease or metastatic carcinoma may produce a myelopathy with sudden onset. Anterior spinal artery infarction is much more common than the posterior artery syndrome because of the difference in collateral supply. Anterior spinal artery occlusion in the cervical area produces tetraplegia, incontinence of urine and feces, and sensory impairment below the lesion which spares proprioception and vibration sense. (**Ref.** 5, pp. 248–249)

16. (E) Moderate fever is frequent at this stage; albuminuria and glycosuria occasionally occur. Retinal hemorrhages, either unilateral or bilateral, may occur and may be accompanied by subhyaloid or vitreous hemorrhage. (**Ref.** 4, pp. 310–313)

17. (A) These data, however, depend to a great extent upon the adequacy of the angiographic study. Multiple aneurysms are often bilateral. (**Ref.** 5, p. 235)

18. (A) At the present time, controversy as to the choice of management continues. Surgical treatment is easily the most popular but it has significant drawbacks, especially with regard to serious treatment—caused morbidity (ie, microsurgically)—caused brain damage. Medical treatment with hypotension has demonstrated continued effectiveness without causing brain damage but it requires the availability of adequate facilities and staff, including neurologists experienced in the use of the method. (**Ref.** 1, pp. 90–99; **Ref.** 2, pp. 180–183; **Ref.** 15, pp. 1357–1361; **Ref.** 16, pp. 7–8)

19. (A) The encouraging results of long-term medical-hypotensive therapy have now been reported by more than one institution. Patients with proven ruptured brain aneurysm treated entirely medically with hypotension have now been followed for more than 30 years without need for any surgery. (**Ref.** 2, pp. 180–183; **Ref.** 10, p. 294; **Ref.** 11, pp. 605–606; **Ref.** 18, p. I-145)

20. (A) Results of medical treatment with hypotension, as noted, are excellent in long-term follow-up as well and, therefore, this medical method has eliminated the so-called annual mortality in non-operated patients. Nevertheless, at the present time, surgical treatment remains the most popular. (Also, see the answer to question #18). More recent developments in Japan of successful obliteration of brain aneurysms (in experimental animals) by simply an intravenous injection of human blood factor XIII has rekindled great interest in the possibility of another completely medical approach, which could also be combined with medical-hypotensive therapy and eliminate the need for surgical treatment. Endovascular treatment with platinum coils is currently under investigation. (**Ref.** 1, pp. 90, 97; **Ref.** 2, pp. 180–183; **Ref.** 15, pp. 1357–1361; **Ref.** 16, pp. 7–8; **Ref.** 17, pp. I-154–155; **Ref.** 28, pp. 1–2)

21. **(A)** This condition is usually silent until the middle years; the process is the same as that found elsewhere in the body. In Caucasians, the carotid artery is responsible for atherothrombotic stroke six to seven times more frequently than is the middle cerebral artery's main trunk; in Asians, the ratio is reversed. **(Ref. 9, p. 2163)**

22. **(C)** These are additional factors believed to contribute to the chance of stroke. Another inflammatory arteriopathy, especially common in Japan, Moyamoya, causes a progressive obliteration of the intracranial carotid arteries. Progressive and stepwise neurologic disability is the rule. **(Ref. 9, p. 2164; Ref. 12, pp. 758–763)**

23. **(C)** Emboli can cause cerebral infarction in the absence of significant cerebral arterial disease. Watershed infarctions especially tend to be hemorrhagic because, with flow restoration, blood to the tissues passes through hypoxic, damaged capillaries. **(Ref. 9, pp. 2162–2164)**

24. **(A)** Emboli from infected material can cause local inflammation as well as infarction. Overall, the declining incidence of rheumatic fever has caused a reduction in mitral stenosis as a cause of thromboembolic stroke. Improved technical diagnostic skills have increased the estimated incidence of cardioembolic stroke. **(Ref. 9, pp. 2090–2092)**

25. **(A)** Involvement of either a venous sinus or of cortical veins can produce infarction; cortical vein involvement is generally extensive and, histologically, one finds an acute inflammatory reaction with neuronal loss. Hemorrhagic infarction may result in the presence of blood in the subarachnoid space. **(Ref. 9, pp. 2165, 2181–2185)**

26. **(B)** Dehydration, head trauma, some blood dyscrasias, and intracerebral hemorrhage are other causes. In the preantibiotic era, retrograde extension of more superficial septic thrombosis was often fatal. Differential diagnosis of cavernous sinus thrombosis includes orbital tumor, meningioma, aneurysm. **(Ref. 9, p. 2185)**

27. (B) The role of hypertension is not as clear as is that of hypotension. Nevertheless, hypertensive encephalopathy is a medical emergency. The long-term prognosis is good if the blood pressure is manageable and other organs are not in end-stage failure. (**Ref.** 9, p. 172)

28. (A) Onset of illness and other non-neurologic features may help. When the stroke has been preceded by transient ischemic attacks, thrombosis becomes more likely. A diagnosis of embolism is also important because the risk of recurrence is high. (**Ref.** 9, pp. 2163–2164; **Ref.** 5, p. 217)

29. (B) The disorder is uncommon but should be considered in patients with infarction who have focal seizures, increased intracranial pressure, or evidence of infection. There may be premonitory headaches and transient ischemic events. Primary sinus thrombosis tends to favor unpaired sinuses and it occurs in association with pregnancy and the puerperium. (**Ref.** 9, p. 2184)

30. (A) In all varieties of cerebral venous thrombosis, some evidence of sepsis is usually found. Since the antibiotic era began, aseptic thrombosis of cerebral veins and sinuses has become more common than the septic variety. The prognosis for aseptic cerebral phlebothrombosis is usually favorable. After optimal treatment of this group of illnesses, prognosis for survival is fairly good but residual neurologic deficits are frequent. (**Ref.** 9, p. 2185)

31. (A) There is often evidence of vascular disease in other areas, a variety of associated diseases and often a previous cerebral infarction. One of the increasingly identified conditions, associated with ischemia, is mitral valve prolapse. A problem is to know when this situation, which occurs asymptomatically in 6% to 8% of normal persons, is a cause of symptoms. (**Ref.** 9, pp. 2162–2165)

32. (B) Spinal tap is an extremely important test for the presence of bleeding or infection. In those cases, it may give crucial information. Traumatic tap must be excluded in the differential diagnosis of bleeding. (**Ref.** 9, pp. 2056, 2170, 2176)

33. (A) The CT or MRI scans are very accurate in ruling in or out intracerebral hemorrhage and brain tumor as causes of neurologic deficit. They have also replaced isotope brain scanning in the study of stroke and threatened stroke. (**Ref.** 9, p. 2170)

34. (B) Cerebral edema probably complicates all cases, but other general changes, such as fever or toxic-metabolic factors, can also cause worsening; without complications, improvement usually begins early. The use of steroids, either alone or with mannitol, has been largely discredited. (**Ref.** 9, p. 2172)

35. (C) In one series, half of the patients who survived the initial cerebral infarction died subsequently of myocardial infarction or cardiac failure. Recurrence of cerebral infarction is common with cerebral emboli of any cause. The prognosis is better in younger patients and in those without hypertension, diabetes mellitus, or severe neurologic defects. (**Ref.** 9, p. 2170)

36. (B) When bleeding occurs, an investigation should be made for a possible additional cause (eg, GI or GU malignancy). In any event, it must be noted that even carefully monitored patients are at risk of serious hemorrhage. Anticoagulation is of no value in completed stroke. (**Ref.** 9, p. 2171)

37. (C) This term more strictly applies to an acute or subacute neurologic disorder due to severe hypertension and renal disease. It is attributed to generalized arteriolar dilatation when cerebral autoregulation is lost. Generalized convulsions may occur. Hypotensive therapy reverses the symptoms and, as usual, should be applied carefully. (**Ref.** 5, pp. 215–216)

38. (E) Non-traumatic intracranial hemorrhage is usually due to ruptured arteries, although veins too may bleed. The two most common causes are bleeding from arterial aneurysm (circle of Willis) and bleeding from arterioles damaged by hypertension or arteriosclerosis. (**Ref.** 9, p. 2173)

39. (A) A change in blood pressure may be the single final event that causes the sac to break. Muscle and elastic tissue defects in the media, possibly of congenital origin, are subjected to the physical effects of pulsatile blood pressure aggravated by turbulence in the circulation through the aneurysm. Aneurysms measuring 2.5 cm in diameter or more are less common and are called giant aneurysms. (**Ref.** 9, pp. 2173–2174)

40. **(B)** Hemorrhage is uncommon but, when it occurs, it is often fatal. Some fusiform aneurysms compress the brain stem. Others mimic cerebellopontine angle tumors; still others simulate pituitary and suprasellar neoplasms. They occur most commonly in the basilar artery. (**Ref.** 9, p. 2174)

41. **(A)** These are produced by septic emboli associated with bacterial endocarditis. The emboli may lead to thromboses or aneurysms. These aneurysms tend to arise in a diagnostically characteristic location along the distal branches of the middle and anterior cerebral arteries rather than at the base. (**Ref.** 9, p. 2174)

42. **(B)** These are tangled vessels, ranging from microscopic to huge, in which arterial blood goes directly to the venous drainage without passing through intervening capillaries. Draining veins may be as large as 1 cm in diameter. The three other types of cerebrovascular malformations are capillary telangiectasia, cavernous angioma, and venous angioma. (**Ref.** 9, p. 2174)

43. **(A)** The role of these changes, as well as that of the microaneurysms of Bouchard and Charcot, is not yet certain. It has been said that the penetrating small arteries develop necrotic degeneration leading to rupturing in some patients, whereas in others a less necrotic process leads to lipohyalinosis with thrombi and lacunes. A ruptured arteriole causes a small hemorrhage, which then compresses surrounding tissues, producing ischemia, which in turn speeds the process of necrotic degeneration of adjacent arterioles, etc. (**Ref.** 9, p. 2178)

44. **(A)** Of all the causes of cerebral hemorrhage, tumors are a very small percentage and yet must be considered in the differential diagnosis. CT or MRI scans and, occasionally, angiography are used in the investigation. Bleeding occurs especially in fast growing malignant gliomas and very vascular secondary tumors. (**Ref.** 9, pp. 2174–2175)

45. (E) Blood becomes a noxious substance, perhaps especially as it hemolyzes and changes into its pigments. Vasospasm is believed to be precipitated by the release, by blood in the subarachnoid space, of vasoactive substances including prostaglandins, serotonin, catecholamines, and methemoglobin. If a patient with a cerebral aneurysm undergoes microsurgical treatment, a postoperative vasospasm can occur, sometimes with catastrophic results. Vasospasm has not significantly affected the results of medical-hypotensive therapy for ruptured brain aneurysms. **(Ref. 9, pp. 2175–2176)**

46. (C) Some report that ischemia and infarcted brain tissue occur in two-thirds of the patients dying from subarachnoid hemorrhage. Vasospasm by angiography usually appears 4 to 10 days after subarachnoid hemorrhage and develops in more than one-third of the patients suffering a ruptured brain aneurysm. **(Ref. 9, pp. 2175–2176)**

47. (C) Some hemorrhages dissect along fiber tracts, with relatively little resultant damage to brain tissue. They may rupture into the ventricles. Relatively few extend directly into the subarachnoid space. In a normotensive, older patient with hemorrhage in the centrum ovale, amyloid angiopathy should be considered. **(Ref. 9, p. 178)**

48. (A) They may also occur during other parts of the acute phase. At the start of hemorrhage, this may be preceded by dizziness or vertigo and vomiting. Neck rigidity is the most common physical sign but may not appear until 12 to 24 hours after onset. **(Ref. 9, p. 2176)**

49. (A) Except for those involving the posterior communicating artery and the "giant" ophthalmic artery aneurysms, a saccular aneurysm generally does not betray its presence prior to rupture. Much less commonly, third nerve palsy is due to a basilar artery aneurysm. Involvement of the third nerve produces impaired adduction of the eye. **(Ref. 9, p. 2176)**

50. (A) Once bleeding has occurred, the clinical picture is the same for aneurysm and arteriovenous malformation. With regard to the bruit, it has been said that skull or orbital bruits may be found in approximately 40% of patients with arteriovenous malformations. Bruit is found only occasionally with berry aneurysms. (**Ref.** 9, p. 2176)

51. **(C)** In about 20% of patients, the hemorrhage is circumscribed and therefore the CSF remains bloodless. The ictus usually occurs when the patient is awake and active, whereas thrombotic obstruction more commonly occurs during sleep. Internal capsular-thalamic lesions may cause fixed downward deviation of the eyes. (**Ref.** 9, pp. 2178–2179)

52. **(C)** If the diagnosis of intracerebellar hemorrhage can be made, surgical treatment may be helpful; however, successful medical treatment of these cases is now also being reported. Careful neurologic clinical monitoring supplemented by CT and MRI scans is used in determining management. Dysphagia must also be watched for. (**Ref.** 9, pp. 2179–2180)

53. **(D)** The color of the supernatant and the white blood cell to red blood cell ratio may depend upon how soon after the bleed lumbar puncture is performed. One should centrifuge one's CSF specimen immediately rather than send it all to the hospital laboratory. CT scan is occasionally falsely negative in subarachnoid hemorrhage. (**Ref.** 9, pp. 2106, 2176)

54. **(A)** Angiography will now demonstrate most aneurysms, arteriovenous malformations, hematomas, and neoplasms. However, a significant number of small lesions escape even the most careful studies. CT and MRI scans complement the angiographic investigation regarding the location of the blood and the cause of the bleeding. (**Ref.** 9, pp. 2176–2177)

55. **(A)** Mortality and morbidity due to surgical treatment are generally too high to permit its routine use. Ligation of feeding vessels, coupled with balloon catheter embolization and the injection of plastic polymers into the vessels of the anomaly, is being carried out in a few centers. Serious complications can occur. (**Ref.** 9, p. 2178)

56. **(B)** A recent controlled study (England) showed that the results of surgical treatment were not as good as those of conservative

treatment. The most satisfactory recoveries occur in patients who have not been submitted to operation. Treatment in general is mostly unsatisfactory in this group of patients. (**Ref.** 9, p. 2180)

57. (D)   This is one of the most common symptoms of vertebrobasilar ischemia; it may be a manifestation of basilar artery migraine. (**Ref.** 9, pp. 2168–2169)

58. (C)   However, if the patient falls suddenly and without warning, "drop attack" is likely. (**Ref.** 9, pp. 2168–2169)

59. (B)   This is another one of the most common symptoms of vertebrobasilar ischemia and may be a manifestation of basilar artery migraine. However, it may also be an important indication of brainstem dysfunction due to any cause whereas vertigo may often have a peripheral etiology. (**Ref.** 9, pp. 2168–2169)

60. (E)   The "crossed syndromes" generally point immediately to brain stem localization. (**Ref.** 9, pp. 2168–2169)

61. (A)   The visual loss frequently involves the entire vision. (**Ref.** 9, pp. 2168–2169)

2

Tumors

DIRECTIONS (Questions 62–67): Each of the questions or incomplete statements below is followed by five suggested answers or completions. Select the ONE lettered answer or completion that is BEST in each case.

---

62. Hemangioblastomas of the cerebellum
  A. may be associated with polycythemia
  B. are seldom associated with renal cysts
  C. tend not to be familial
  D. are usually solid
  E. generally produce symptoms in the first two decades of life

63. The two most common sources of metastasis to the brain are
  A. breast and lung
  B. lung and colon
  C. colon and rectum
  D. rectum and nasal sinuses
  E. uterus and ovary

64. The cranial nerve most often involved in neurofibromatosis is the
  A. oculomotor
  B. trigeminal
  C. facial
  D. vagus
  E. hypoglossal

65. The most important false localizing sign of intracranial tumor is
  A. anosognosia
  B. homonymous hemianopsia
  C. oculomotor palsy
  D. abducens palsy
  E. mydraisis

66. Meningiomas seldom
  A. are extracerebral
  B. invade the skull
  C. are infratentorial
  D. occur along venous sinuses
  E. form columns or whorls

67. In the investigation for possible acoustic neuroma
  A. the CSF protein is elevated in at least three-quarters of the cases unless the tumor is small
  B. a 2-mm enlargement of the internal auditory meatus may be disregarded
  C. caloric abnormalities and a progressive pattern of involvement of the seventh, fifth, and twelfth cranial nerves are important
  D. choked discs are seen early
  E. posterior fossa myelography is not indicated

DIRECTIONS (Questions 68–72): The group of questions below consists of lettered headings followed by a list of numbered words or statements. For each numbered word or statement, select the ONE lettered heading that is most closely associated with it. Each lettered heading may be selected once, more than once, or not at all.

A. Most malignant
B. Most often contain calcium
C. Parinaud's syndrome
D. Relatively radiosensitive posterior fossa tumor of childhood
E. Relatively radioresistant posterior fossa tumor of childhood

68. Pinealoma

69. Glioblastoma multiforme

70. Medulloblastoma

71. Oligodendroglioma

72. Ependymoma

DIRECTIONS (Questions 73–97): Each set of lettered headings below is followed by a list of numbered words or phrases. For each numbered word or phrase select

A. if the item is associated with A only
B. if the item is associated with B only
C. if the item is associated with both A and B
D. if the item is associated with neither A nor B

Questions 73–82:

A. Glioblastoma multiforme
B. Oligodendroglioma
C. Both
D. Neither

73. A small percentage of the gliomas

74. Most frequently located in cerebral hemispheres

75. Areas of cystic degeneration are uncommon

76. Hemorrhage areas are uncommon

77. Seed into CSF, causing tumors in other regions of the nervous system

78. Amenable to complete surgical removal

79. Plain skull x-rays frequently show characteristic flecks of calcium

80. Most often are rapidly fatal, leading to death in one year

81. Very cellular, with cells uniform in size and shape

82. Occasionally spread to the opposite hemisphere by way of the corpus callosum

Questions 83–97:

    A. Sphenoid ridge meningioma
    B. Olfactory groove or suprasellar meningioma
    C. Both
    D. Neither

83. Exophthalmos

84. Primary optic atrophy

85. Extraocular palsies

86. Numbness of the brow

87. Unilateral anosmia

88. Foster Kennedy syndrome

89. Arise from tuberculum sellae or diaphragm of the sella

90. Subdivided into two groups

91. Vivid visual hallucinations

92. Meningioma en plaque

93. Olfactory hallucinations are common

94. Mental changes

95. Syndrome similar to that of pituitary adenoma

96. Gustatory hallucinations are common

97. Nystagmus

Answers and Discussion

62. (A) Most commonly, headache and papilledema are noted; there may or may not be signs or symptoms of cerebellar dysfunction. The second most common site of hemangioblastomas is the spinal cord. Most often, young and middle-aged adults are afflicted. Von Hippel-Lindau disease includes, in addition, multiple angiomatoses of the retina plus cysts of the kidney and pancreas. (**Ref.** 5, pp. 333–334)

63. (A) Almost any malignancy may metastasize to the brain, but in about 60% of the cases, the lung or breast is the source of the primary tumor. Melanomas, choriocarcinomas, and hypernephromas are associated with a high incidence of tumor hemorrhage. In about 10% of the cases, no primary tumor can be found. (**Ref.** 5, pp. 341–343)

64. (D) The trigeminal nerve is said to be the second most often involved; an entity in which bilateral acoustic nerve involvement is the only manifestation of the disease has also been reported. Visual compromise may occur as a result of glaucoma, buphthalmos, optic nerve gliosis, and uveal coat involvement. (**Ref.** 5, pp. 365–367)

65. (D) This may be unilateral or bilateral. In addition, bilateral extensor plantar reflexes or bilateral grasp reflexes may result from interference with the function of the cerebral hemispheres by distension of the ventricles in hydrocephalus. (**Ref.** 4, pp. 230–231)

66. (C) They are found especially at the superior sagittal sinus, sphenoid ridge, hemisphere convexities, and suprasellar region. In their invasion of the bone, they provoke a characteristic hyperostosis. **(Ref. 4, p. 225)**

67. (A) If the initial symptoms are not referable to the auditory nerve, and if the CSF and caloric tests are normal, acoustic neuroma is unlikely. Brain stem auditory evoked responses (BAER) are very sensitive. More recently, magnetic resonance has replaced myelography in at least some instances. **(Ref. 5, pp. 288–290)**

68. (C) This tumor also frequently causes dilated, fixed pupils and impaired hearing. The most common type is the germ cell tumor, especially the germinoma; the next most common is the astrocytoma. Parinaud's syndrome includes paralysis of upward gaze, convergence, and irregular pupillary responses to light and accommodation. **(Ref. 5, pp. 314–318)**

69. (A) This constitutes about one-third of all gliomas. This rapidly growing tumor occasionally grows in the opposite hemisphere through the corpus callosum ("butterfly glioma"). **(Ref. 5, pp. 298–300)**

70. (D) This metastasizes to the cerebrum, the spinal cord, and even to other parts of the body. In children, these tumors are commonly in the midline, arising from the posterior vermis; in adults, they are frequently seen in the cerebellar hemispheres. **(Ref. 5, pp. 304–305)**

71. (B) This occurs in the cerebral hemispheres and the cerebral ventriclesatients may have symptoms, especially seizures, for many years before the presence of a mass lesion becomes obvious; on the other hand, these tumors may have a malignant course. **(Ref. 5, p. 303)**

72. (E) This is difficult to remove surgically and is relatively malignant. It is commonly seen in the fourth ventricle, frequently obstructs the cerebrospinal fluid pathways, and may cause focal symptoms. **(Ref. 5, p. 305)**

73. (B) These comprise less than 5% of all gliomas. The average survival period for this tumor was given, in an older study, as 66 months. (**Ref.** 5, p. 303)

74. (C) Oligodendrogliomas can also occur in the third ventricle; glioblastoma multiforme can occur anywhere in the central nervous system. It is found especially in the frontal lobe of young adults. (**Ref.** 5, p. 303)

75. (B) These tumors are firm in consistency. Microscopically, there are many cells that are uniform in size and shape, evenly spaced, or in a loose meshwork. (**Ref.** 5, p. 303)

76. (B) These tumors are more often circumscribed than are the rapidly growing gliomas. The tumor's course is somewhat unpredictable and does not always correlate with the histologic appearance. (**Ref.** 5, p. 303)

77. (A) These are the most rapidly growing gliomas. In autopsy series, these tumors are found to have spread through the subarachnoid spaces in about 35% of the cases. (**Ref.** 5, pp. 298–300)

78. (D) Surgery may make the patients much worse. Surgical authors may feel that surgical treatment must be used (followed by radiotherapy) for both of these tumors; not everyone agrees. (**Ref.** 5, pp. 298–303)

79. (B) About 50% of these tumors (at postmortem) have calcium flecks. Whether the patient is treated medically or surgically, CT or nuclear magnetic resonance are useful laboratory tests in following the subsequent course, along with periodic evaluation. (**Ref.** 5, p. 303)

80. (A) They invade large portions of the hemisphere. Clinically, one sees a combination of signs of increased intracranial pressure and focal neurologic abnormalities. (**Ref.** 5, pp. 298–300)

81. (B) Nuclei are round, with much chromatin, and are surrounded by a faint cytoplasmic halo. Instead of the frequently found slow course, a malignant course with local or even systemic dissemination may take place. (**Ref.** 5, p. 303)

82. (A) Cells are of many sizes and shapes; mitotic figures and bizarre giant cells are common. This tumor is localized more frequently in the frontal and temporal lobes; occasionally it is multicentric. (**Ref.** 5, pp. 298–300)

83. (A) This is associated with hyperostosis. Exophthalmos occurs in either the pterional or the clinoidal type. (**Ref.** 5, pp. 294–296)

84. (C) In the clinoidal type, the presenting symptom is often unilateral visual failure. The optic nerve is often compressed or surrounded early. (**Ref.** 5, pp. 294–296)

85. (A) These are homolateral. They occur when the superior orbital fissure is involved. (**Ref.** 5, pp. 294–296)

86. (A) Due to involvement of the ophthalmic branch of the trigeminal nerve. This occurs in the clinoidal type. (**Ref.** 5, pp. 294–296)

87. (B) A common early finding in olfactory groove tumors. These arise from the cribriform and ethmoid regions. They may become very large. (**Ref.** 5, pp. 294–296)

88. (C) A frequent finding when the tumor remains localized to one side. Dementia may result from compression of the anterior cerebral arteries and frontal lobes. (**Ref.** 5, pp. 294–296)

89. (B) Those that arise from the tuberculum sellae may show a hyperostotic tuberculum on x-ray. In addition, a characteristic angiographic picture is found (enlarged, penetrating ophthalmic artery branches). (**Ref.** 5, pp. 294–296)

90. (A) Inner sphenoid ridge or clinoidal type and outer sphenoid ridge or pterional type. The pterional type may be of the globoid or the en plaque variety. (**Ref.** 5, pp. 294–296)

91. (A) The patient can often describe, in detail, people and objects in his hallucinations. Seizures may occur. (**Ref.** 5, pp. 294–296)

92. (A) A flat tumor, one of two types of outer sphenoid ridge tumors. This type of outer sphenoid ridge tumor occurs most frequently in women. **(Ref.** 5, pp. 294–296)

93. (A) Convulsive seizures here are more often generalized than Jacksonian. Seizures are associated with the outer sphenoid ridge location. **(Ref.** 5, pp. 294–296)

94. (C) Areas of involvement include the frontal lobes. This occurs either via direct parenchymal compression or by interference with its blood supply. **(Ref.** 5, pp. 294–296)

95. (B) The group that arises from the tuberculum sellae and compresses the optic chiasm. They may also be mistaken for giant carotid artery aneurysms. **(Ref.** 5, pp. 294–296)

96. (A) These occur in both groups of sphenoid ridge meningiomas. The pterional type of tumor is easier to remove if the infiltrated dura can be surgically resected. **(Ref.** 5, pp. 294–296)

97. (D) This is generally a sign of brain stem dysfunction. Posterior fossa meningiomas may cause this (eg, in the cerebellopontine angle); they mimic acoustic nerve tumors. **(Ref.** 5, pp. 294–296)

3

Trauma

DIRECTIONS (Questions 98–118): Each of the questions or incomplete statements below is followed by suggested answers or completions. Select the ONE lettered answer or completion that is BEST in each case.

98. In neoplastic or disc compression of the cauda equina, the first symptom is usually
    A. paresthesia
    B. pain
    C. paralysis
    D. Babinski sign
    E. none of the above

99. After head trauma
   A. post-traumatic amnesia usually lasts longer than retrograde amnesia
   B. retrograde amnesia usually lasts longer than post-traumatic amnesia
   C. headache occurs in approximately 50% of the patients upon recovery of consciousness
   D. Hutchinson's pupil may occur, usually first on the side opposite the lesion
   E. Hutchinson's pupil may be seen, beginning with dilatation

100. The carpal tunnel syndrome
   A. usually affects the musculocutaneous nerve
   B. usually does not affect the median nerve
   C. has occurred in myxedema, acromegaly, or pregnancy
   D. does not cause thenar atrophy
   E. affects the radial nerve

101. The most common cause of bilateral lower motor neuron hypoglossal paralysis is
   A. polio
   B. progressive bulbar palsy
   C. metastatic disease
   D. diabetes
   E. none of the above

102. The most common cause of unilateral lower motor neuron hypoglossal paralysis is
   A. thrombosis of the posterior inferior cerebellar artery
   B. tumor
   C. trauma
   D. meningoencephalitis
   E. none of the above

103. With a herniated disc, if the deep tendon reflexes were intact and the peronei were weak, one would locate the lesion at the root
   A. L2
   B. L3

C. L4
D. L5
E. S1

104. Peripheral neuropathy in patients with visc   is
    A. more commonly a purely sensory disorder y
    B. more commonly a purely motor disorder
    C. more commonly a purely autonomic disorder
    D. more commonly a mixed sensory-motor disorder
    E. more commonly, paresthesias are not marked and generally
       are asymmetric

105. Subdural hematoma does *not*
    A. present with convulsions, either unilateral or generalized
    B. have xanthochromic cerebrospinal fluid
    C. have remissions and exacerbations
    D. invariably produce ipsilateral hemiplegia
    E. frequently produce a Babinski sign

106. Bell's palsy
    A. is attributable to non-suppurative inflammation of the facial
       nerve
    B. does not occur in herpes zoster
    C. is most common in elderly males
    D. is most common in elderly females
    E. frequently results in permanent severe paralysis

107. Obstetrical paralyses of the brachial plexus generally
    A. are the upper arm type
    B. are the lower arm type
    C. involve the total plexus
    D. produce marked sensory dysfunction
    E. produce vasomotor dysfunction

108. The most common causes of lesions of the cauda equina are
    A. trauma, tumor, and inflammation
    B. tumor, vascular malformations, and inflammation
    C. metabolic and toxic diseases
    D. congenital malformations and occlusive vascul
    E. trauma and bony anomalies

.or nerve were injured in severe labor, one would ex-

.gesia of the anterior aspect of the thigh without accom-
ying motor deficit
ontinence
⊃o symptoms
severe impairment of walking
impairment of crossing the legs

110. Partial or complete recovery from Bell's palsy
    A.   occurs in approximately 50% of cases
    B.   may be complicated by "crocodile" tears
    C.   may be complicated by facial spasms that are not seen in pa-
        tients who have not had a facial nerve lesion
    D.   does not depend on the severity of the lesion
    E.   is likely even when the nerve is anatomically sectioned

111. Meralgia paresthetica
    A.   is frequently treated by splitting the fascia lata
    B.   usually disappears after approximately three weeks
    C.   is usually unilateral
    D.   affects women more than men
    E.   none of the above

112. Femoral nerve injury
    A.   is common
    B.   permits walking on level ground with the leg extended
    C.   does not affect walking uphill
    D.   does not affect climbing stairs
    E.   none of the above

113. The 11th cranial nerve
    A.   is unaffected by demyelination in the medulla
    B.   is unaffected peripherally by inflammation
    C.   supplies muscles that are frequently involved in myotonia
        atrophica
    ⊃.   is not involved in necrotic occipital bone processes
        none of the above

114. Following a head injury, the elec
ally   phalogra'
    A. go through a phase of slowing a.
    B. become unusually responsive to hy
    C. show evidence of focal damage to
    D. show suppression of electrical ac.
        weeks after the injury
    E. none of the above

115. Lesions of the nucleus ambiguus
    A. if unilateral, produce dysarthria and dysphagia
    B. produce dysphagia if the lesion involves the upper part of the
        nucleus
    C. produce dysarthria if the lesion involves the lower part of the
        nucleus
    D. cause ipsilateral uvula deviation on phonation
    E. none of the above

116. Bilateral lesions of the nucleus ambiguus
    A. are rare except in amyotrophic lateral sclerosis
    B. cause complete aphonia only rarely
    C. cause complete aphagia only rarely
    D. cause serious autonomic dysfunction
    E. none of the above

117. Extradural hemorrhage
    A. always affects the middle meningeal artery
    B. is often bilateral
    C. almost invariably has a lucid interval
    D. is a relatively common complication of head injury
    E. none of the above

118. Extradural hemorrhage
    A. usually is located over the hemisphere convexity in the mid-
        dle fossa
    B. usually produces bloody cerebrospinal fluid
    C. is generally followed by a lucid interval of several days
    D. produces contralateral pupillary dilatation
    E. usually produces homolateral hemiplegia

DIRECTIONS (Q̃s 119–123): The set of lettered headings below is followed̃e select list of numbered words or phrases. For each numbered word q̃s associated with A only

A. if thẽ is associated with A only
B. if thẽ is associated with B only
C. if thẽem is associated with both A and B
D. i'tʰ item is associated with neither A nor B

A. Electrical injuries
B. Decompression sickness
C. Boᵗʰ
D. Neither

119. Convulsions

120. Most serious complication is paralysis due to myelopathy

121. Death due to respiratory arrest or ventricular fibrillation

122. Marcus Gunn phenomenon

123. Gunn pupil

Answers and Discussion

98. (B) Bladder and bowel dysfunction, generally retention, tend to occur late when the lowest sacral roots are compressed. The external genitalia become anesthetic. When atrophic paralysis occurs, it most frequently involves the muscles below the knee. **(Ref. 4, p. 372)**

99. (A) Retrograde amnesia often lasts only for seconds whereas post-traumatic amnesia may last for minutes to weeks. Retrograde amnesia may be prolonged when there is selective bitemporal brain damage. Hutchinson's pupil begins ipsilaterally to the side of the lesion. At first, it constricts and then it dilates with failure to react to light. **(Ref. 4, pp. 171, 277)**

100. (C) This also occurs with wrist fractures and arthritis. The spontaneous variety is frequently bilateral but often begins in one hand several months or longer before it starts in the other. **(Ref. 4, p. 411)**

101. (B) Fasciculations are prominent during active degeneration. The medullary nuclei may also be attacked in bulbar polio. **(Ref. 4, p. 86)**

102. (B) Unilateral lower motor neuron lesions of the tongue are uncommon; they may occur at the nucleus or at the nerve fibers between medulla and hypoglossal canal. Unilateral paralysis of the tongue does not impair articulation. It is not part of the posterior inferior cerebellar artery syndrome. (**Ref.** 4, p. 86)

103. **(D)**   Pain would involve the lateral aspect of the leg. Pain is often increased by coughing, sneezing, stooping, sitting, and walking. There may be individual variation in terms of which posture aggravates the pain most severely. The other commonly affected root, S1, causes impairment of the ankle jerk. (**Ref.** 4, p. 398)

104. **(D)**   Clinically, subacute evolution of the peripheral neuropathy is characteristic. Paresthesias are prominent and usually symmetric. (**Ref.** 5, pp. 876–880)

105. **(D)**   Hemiplegia may be present and may be either ipsilateral or contralateral to the lesion. (**Ref.** 5, pp. 378–382)

106. **(A)**   Hyperacusis is attributed to involvement of the stapedius. Bell's palsy occurs most often in young adults and most patients obtain nearly complete recovery. (**Ref.** 4, pp. 67–68)

107. **(A)**   Either the upper or lower arm type may occur, but usually it is the upper (Erb-Duchenne); atrophy is marked. This also occurs after falls. The muscles paralyzed are those innervated by C5 segment. (**Ref.** 4, p. 405)

108. **(A)**   The tumors are often malignant and may arise within the spinal canal or grow into it from the bones. Trophic symptoms may occur in the lower limbs, besides the pain, weakness, and sphincter dysfunction. (**Ref.** 4, pp. 372–373)

109. **(E)**   Thigh external rotation and adduction are weakened; hypalgesia is found at the middle, medial part of the thigh. Knee joint pain can be caused by pelvic involvement of the geniculate branch of the obturator. (**Ref.** 5, p. 436)

110. **(B)**   Synkinesias involving either the upper or lower half of the musculature are also common. If recovery is complete, there is no apparent difference between the two sides of the face either at rest or in motion. Anatomical sectioning of the nerve makes chances for complete or even partial recovery remote. (**Ref.** 5, pp. 422–424)

111. (C) The course is variable; removal of constricting garments may help; some advise a decrease in walking. Although it has a long, superficial course, which therefore exposes it to various forms of trauma, in most cases there is no history of trauma to explain the onset of symptoms. **(Ref.** 5, p. 437)

112. (B) In the upright position, the leg is kept extended by the tensor fasciae femoris and the gracilis; even slight flexion while walking causes the limb to give way. The quadriceps reflex is lost on the affected side, and some cutaneous sensation is impaired. **(Ref.** 5, p. 437)

113. (C) The nucleus may also be damaged by inflammatory or degenerative disease, and the peripheral part by extramedullary tumors or by processes in meninges and occipital bone. Myasthenia gravis and polymyositis frequently involve muscles supplied by this nerve. **(Ref.** 5, p. 428)

114. (D) The hypersensitivity to hyperventilation and the focal abnormal activity may persist for weeks or months after the injury. The importance of serial EEG has declined. **(Ref.** 5, pp. 374–375)

115. (A) The longitudinal extent of the nucleus in the medulla permits different kinds of effects of lesions. The ipsilateral palatal reflex is absent. Lower nuclear lesions cause dysphagia; upper nuclear lesions cause dysarthria. **(Ref.** 5, p. 427)

116. (A) This is contrasted to the situation involving unilateral lesions, where the dysphagia and dysarthria are rarely severe. Symptoms of autonomic dysfunction do not occur in unilateral dorsal motor nucleus lesions; however, bilateral lesions of that nucleus are life-threatening. **(Ref.** 5, p. 427)

117. (E) In about 15% of the cases, the bleeding is from a dural sinus. Occasionally, the hemorrhage may be confined to the anterior fossa, possibly due to tearing of an anterior meningeal artery. Extradural hemorrhage is a relatively rare complication of head injury. **(Ref.** 5, pp. 376–378)

118. (A) The lucid interval is often absent. The initial loss of consciousness is due to concussion. The CSF is usually clear, but may be bloody if there has also been contusion or laceration of the brain. **(Ref.** 5, pp. 376–378)

119. (C) In an acute state of electrical injuries, these often accompany loss of consciousness. In decompression sickness, divers' neurologic lesions tend to affect the spinal cord, whereas flyers are more likely to experience cerebral damage. **(Ref.** 5, pp. 445–446)

120. (B) Gas bubbles cause ischemic areas, especially in the white material of the thoracic cord. Upper lumbar cord segments are less often affected, and lower cervical cord segments are least often affected. **(Ref.** 5, pp. 445–446)

121. (A) Immediate treatment is needed to save the patient's life and to prevent further damage to the nervous system. Peripheral nerves also may be damaged, but they are injured by direct effects of the current. **(Ref.** 5, pp. 445–446)

122. (D) Unrelated eyelid-jaw reflex. A partially ptotic eyelid elevates on jaw movement, especially lateral jaw movement. **(Ref.** 5, pp. 445–446)

123. (D) Unrelated pupillary light reflex abnormality. This is demonstrable by the swinging flashlight test. **(Ref.** 5, pp. 445–446)

4

Infections

DIRECTIONS (Questions 124–153): Each of the questions or incomplete statements below is followed by five suggested answers or completions. Select the ONE lettered answer or completion that is BEST in each case.

---

124. General features of brain abscess include:

  A. headache, drowsiness, and confusion; headache is almost always insidious in onset, and fever is present in 90% of cases
  B. papilledema, usually noted early
  C. sixth nerve palsy; less often, third nerve palsy
  D. low mortality today, with antimicrobial therapy and microsurgery
  E. in most cases, a 2-week course of antibiotic therapy is sufficient

125. In the examination of CSF, hypoglycorrhachia does not occur in

  A. tuberculous meningitis
  B. mycotic meningitis
  C. carcinomatous meningitis
  D. sympathetic meningitis
  E. bacterial meningitis

126. In cryptococcal meningoencephalitis
   A. sugar may be reduced, but this effect may be somewhat off-set if the patient is diabetic
   B. polymorphonuclear cells usually predominate
   C. organisms can be recovered by embryonated egg inoculation
   D. CSF pressure is typically normal
   E. Indian ink is helpful; the skin test is negative

127. In tuberculous meningoencephalitis
   A. the pressure may be low in later stages
   B. actual tubercles can seldom be demonstrated in the meninges
   C. the white blood cell count frequently exceeds 1,000/mm^3
   D. CSF protein is usually normal
   E. lymphocytes predominate early

128. In the acute stage of bacterial meningitis, cranial nerve palsies
   A. most often include blindness and facial palsy
   B. less often include ocular movement dysfunction, deafness, and labyrinthine disturbance
   C. are probably due to meningeal exudate, except that the eighth cranial nerve may suffer direct toxic or infectious damage
   D. generally tend to persist even after recovery from the meningitis
   E. include the eighth cranial nerve less often if the organism is *Neisseria meningitidis*

129. Cryptococcic meningitis does not
   A. occur more readily with immunosuppressive treatment
   B. occur more readily in leukemia, lymphoma, and diabetes
   C. occur more readily in sarcoidosis
   D. occur more readily in certain occupations
   E. occur at some ages more often than at others

130. Sarcoidosis
   A. especially involves blood vessels at the convexity of the brain
   B. causes diabetes insipidus and amblyopia due to involvement of the hypothalamus and optic chiasm
   C. does not usually cause hydrocephalus

    D. causes seizures but not cerebellar ataxia
    E. produces neuropathy but not myopathy

131. Viral encephalitis
    A. characteristically features alterations of consciousness
    B. seldom causes seizures
    C. usually does not produce focal signs
    D. often produces a parkinsonian tremor
    E. produces hyperthermia; poikilothermia does not occur

132. Brain abscess
    A. has decreased significantly over the past 20 years
    B. is due to otitic infection in more than one-third of the cases
    C. is common in infancy, especially in patients with congenital heart disease
    D. presents most often with drowsiness and nausea; later, confusion occurs
    E. infrequently involves the temporal lobe

133. In Creutzfeldt-Jakob disease
    A. affected individuals may expect to live for approximately 8 to 10 years
    B. the spinal cord is involved
    C. myoclonus does not occur
    D. attempts at transmission to primates have not yet been successful
    E. the EEG characteristically shows spikes early in the course of the disease

134. The pathologic findings in fatal cases of meningococcal meningitis
    A. are very similar to those of all other types of purulent meningitis
    B. frequently include parenchymal abscesses
    C. may include hydrocephalus but not disseminated intravascular coagulation
    D. continue to include a high percentage of complications
    E. continue to include a high percentage of sequelae

135. At the onset, a case of bacterial meningitis would be most likely to show
   A. systemic symptoms and signs
   B. cranial bruit
   C. central scotoma
   D. bitemporal hemianopsia
   E. fasciculations

136. The neurologic manifestations of early bacterial meningitis include
   A. stiff neck and hypertension
   B. Kernig and Brudzinski signs
   C. photophobia and papilledema
   D. bradycardia
   E. hypothermia

137. Influenzal meningitis differs from other types in that
   A. it occurs almost exclusively in infants and young children
   B. the organism can seldom be cultured
   C. neurologic complications do not occur
   D. the CSF changes are distinctive
   E. the clinical pattern is distinctive

138. One of the important complications of influenzal meningitis is
   A. anosognosia
   B. bulimia
   C. diabetes insipidus
   D. subdural effusion
   E. teleopsia

139. Sequelae of tuberculous meningitis include
   A. calcification of the basilar meninges and especially the parenchyma
   B. deafness and convulsions
   C. blindness but not quadriplegia
   D. hemiplegia but not paraplegia
   E. IQ of less than 80, but rarely

140. The neurologic complications of sarcoidosis include
  - **A.** facial palsy (including taste fibers), provided parotitis has occurred
  - **B.** optic neuritis, in addition to uveitis, but not optic atrophy
  - **C.** subacute meningitis, but without chronic adhesive arachnoiditis
  - **D.** visual field defects and diabetes insipidus
  - **E.** peripheral neuropathy, motor type only

141. Behçet's syndrome
  - **A.** produces supratentorial and infratentorial symptoms
  - **B.** does not lead to complete blindness
  - **C.** does not produce an organic mental syndrome
  - **D.** occasionally produces a positive Kveim-Siltzbach test
  - **E.** characteristically has a steadily progressive course

142. An aseptic meningeal reaction
  - **A.** is a condition that may indicate a serious infection
  - **B.** may lead to CSF that appears purulent; sugar content is decreased
  - **C.** may be seen after the introduction of drugs into the CSF; protein is normal
  - **D.** causes no significant rise in CSF pressure
  - **E.** does not occur in brain tumor

143. Cerebral subdural abscess is differentiated from extradural abscess in that
  - **A.** the latter leads to nuchal rigidity
  - **B.** the latter is less likely to produce focal signs
  - **C.** the former leads to a less acute illness
  - **D.** the former is painless
  - **E.** sinus thrombosis more often accompanies extradural abscess

144. Spinal epidural abscess
  - **A.** is relatively common
  - **B.** is unaccompanied by fever
  - **C.** is unaccompanied by headache
  - **D.** occurs mainly by direct extension
  - **E.** does not occur by perforating wounds or by direct extension

145. The most common site of spinal epidural abscess is
- **A.** cervical
- **B.** thoracic
- **C.** lumbar
- **D.** sacral
- **E.** equal in all

146. The differential diagnosis of spinal epidural abscess includes
- **A.** primary but not metastatic tumor
- **B.** Andersen disease
- **C.** Sotas syndrome
- **D.** acute or subacute meningitis
- **E.** Sly syndrome

147. A frequent cause of brain abscess is
- **A.** pneumococcus
- **B.** meningococcus
- **C.** *Hemophilus influenzae*
- **D.** staphylococcus
- **E.** *Entamoeba histolytica*

148. Progressive multifocal leukoencephalopathy
- **A.** produces loss of axis cylinders, with little loss of myelin
- **B.** produces hemiplegia and cranial neuropathies
- **C.** is not associated with myelitis
- **D.** has not been reported in the apparent absence of a primary disease
- **E.** has not been associated with JC virus

149. Infectious mononucleosis
- **A.** invades the nervous system in approximately 20% to 25% of cases
- **B.** produces lymphocytic pleocytosis in the CSF without neurologic symptoms or signs
- **C.** frequently produces headache, stiff neck, and delirium
- **D.** commonly causes optic neuritis
- **E.** commonly causes facial neuritis

150. In infectious mononucleosis
  A. the prognosis is excellent even in cases with respiratory paralysis
  B. serologic tests for syphilis in the CSF may be positive
  C. the CSF protein level is markedly increased
  D. antibody responses to EB virus antigens is helpful
  E. the CSF sugar is decreased

151. Mucormycosis
  A. is usually a complication of diabetes but not of leukemia
  B. follows the usage of antibiotics and steroids
  C. causes thromboses of the ophthalmic and internal carotid arteries, but not of the veins
  D. produces a meningoencephalitis; culture of rhizopus is diagnostic
  E. when invading the nervous system, it increases mortality to 50% to 60%

152. Leprosy
  A. commonly affects the sixth and seventh cranial nerves
  B. produces early proprioceptive loss and sensory dissociation
  C. produces a progressive peroneal palsy
  D. bacilli have not been found in the spinal cord or brain
  E. in the neural form, it proceeds slowly but is invariably fatal

153. Manifestations of acute bacterial meningitis
  A. include seizures only rarely at the onset
  B. include a "meningeal cry" in children
  C. do not include hyporeflexia
  D. include focal signs, especially at the onset
  E. include neuropathies, especially at the onset

DIRECTIONS (Questions 154–156): The group of questions below consists of a list of lettered headings followed by a list of numbered words, phrases, or statements. For each numbered word, phrase, or statement, select the ONE lettered heading that is most closely associated with it. Each lettered heading may be selected once, more than once, or not at all.

Questions 154–158:

    A. Heterophil antigen
    B. Virus recoverable from saliva
    C. Virus recoverable from stool, throat washings, or CSF
    D. Virus recoverable from CSF or blood
    E. Frei test

154. Rabies

155. Infectious mononucleosis

156. Lymphogranuloma venereum

157. Coxsackie

158. Lymphocytic choriomeningitis

Questions 159–166:

    A. Antirabies vaccination
    B. *Plasmodium falciparium*
    C. *Rickettsia rickettsii*
    D. Encephalitis lethargica
    E. *R. mooseri*
    F. Antitetanus vaccination
    G. Progressive multifocal leukoencephalopathy
    H. Cat-scratch fever

159. Virus, possibly in the Papova group, with giant astrocytes, and a decrease in the number of oligodendroglia

160. In the acute state, has produced almost every known neurological sign and symptom; practically extinct now

161. Lymphadenopathy, positive skin test, no fatalities or serious sequelae thus far reported

162. Clinical picture of Landry's paralysis

163. Paralysis of muscles innervated by axillary and long thoracic nerves

164. Rash, pains, headache, stiff neck, positive Weil-Felix test, flea-borne

165. Tick-borne, rash at more distal parts of extremities, positive Weil-Felix test

166. Transfusion, chloroquine, quinine—a medical emergency

DIRECTIONS (Questions 167–171): The set of lettered headings below is followed by a list of numbered words or phrases. For each numbered word or phrase select

   A. if the item is associated with A only
   B. if the item is associated with B only
   C. if the item is associated with both A and B
   D. if the item is associated with neither A nor B

   A. Infectious polyneuritis
   B. Poliomyelitis
   C. Both
   D. Neither

167. Albuminocytologic dissociation

168. Asymmetric paralysis

169. Inability to alpha-oxidize injected phytanic acid

170. Neuropathy superimposed upon history of arthralgia, skin eruptions, fever, albuminuria, and possibly cerebral symptoms

171. First division of the Gasserian ganglion and intercostal dermatomes are most affected

Answers and Discussion

124. (C) The illness may be acute, systemically; yet, approximately one-third of the patients remain afebrile. Progress of the pathologic process does not correlate well with the clinical course. Symptoms of acute infection are often lacking unless the focus giving rise to the abscess is still active. (**Ref.** 9, pp. 2182–2183)

125. (D) This may be due to high metabolic activity of rapidly growing cells, phagocytosis, and reduced glucose transport in the situations where it does occur. Exceptionally, and without explanation, the aseptic meningeal reactions of systemic lupus erythematosus may be accompanied by low CSF sugar values. (**Ref.** 5, pp. 83–84)

126. (A) Organisms are found via the India ink preparation and on culture with Sabouraud's medium. The India ink preparation is positive in only about 50% of cases of crytococcal (torula) meningitis, whereas CSF cultures are eventually positive in about 95%. (**Ref.** 9, p. 1845)

127. (A) Organisms may be found via pellicle smear, guinea pig inoculation, or by culture; tubercles are demonstrable in the meninges in almost every case. The CSF shows high protein, low sugar, and a moderate number of leukocytes. Early, the latter are neutrophilic; later, lymphocytic. (**Ref.** 9, p. 1691)

128. (C) Cranial nerve palsies are common; some workers estimate that 5% to 20% of patients will develop them. The cranial nerves most often affected are the third, fourth, sixth, and seventh. Hearing impairment has more than one cause. (**Ref.** 9, p. 1606)

129. (**D**)   Fungi are more likely to invade the nervous system when host defenses are impaired. Therefore, when mycotic meningitis is found, the possible presence of an additional disease should be considered. Neutropenia appears to confer no additional risk. Clinical manifestations relate in part to host defense status; patients with AIDS have few symptoms or signs despite far-advanced infections. (**Ref.** 9, p. 1845)

130. (**B**)   Almost any part of the nervous system may be involved by sarcoidosis. Diagnosis depends upon other clinical data and/or tissue biopsy. The CSF often shows pleocytosis, increased protein, and, rarely, low glucose. (**Ref.** 9, pp. 453–454)

131. (**A**)   In addition, spinal cord involvement can lead to flaccid paralysis. Increased intracranial pressure can cause third and sixth nerve palsies. Some patients develop hemiparesis, visual symptoms or sensory loss. (**Ref.** 9, p. 2193)

132. (**B**)   Brain abscess results from extension from adjacent foci or from hematogenous spread; congenital heart disease is an important predisposing factor. Otogenic brain abscesses are usually located in the temporal lobe or cerebellum. (**Ref.** 9, p. 2181)

133. (**B**)   The main pathologic changes occur in the cortex, basal ganglia, and spinal cord. Inadvertent human-to-human transmission has been reported following corneal transplantation and the use of inadequately sterilized stereotactic brain electrodes. The course is rapid, with death occurring usually within a few months to a year. (**Ref.** 5, pp. 128–129)

134. (**A**)   The pathology, symptomatology, and course are all similar, regardless of the causative organism; basilar adhesions block the flow of CSF from the fourth ventricle and cause hydrocephalus. In acute fulminating cases, death may occur before there are any significant pathologic changes in the nervous system. (**Ref.** 5, pp. 63–64)

135. **(A)** Cranial nerve palsies and focal neurologic signs usually don't occur until several days after the onset of the infection. The systemic picture includes chills, fever, headaches, nausea, vomiting, back pain, stiff neck, and prostration. (**Ref.** 5, p. 64)

136. **(B)** At the onset, irritability is noted, and, in children, a "meningeal cry." With worsening, clouded sensorium, stupor, or coma may develop. (**Ref.** 5, p. 64)

137. **(A)** Ninety percent occur before the age of five years; the organisms are cultured from blood and CSF; complications occur especially in the untreated. The mortality rate in untreated cases in infants is over 90%. (**Ref.** 5, pp. 66–67)

138. **(D)** Subdural tapping through the fontanelles usually helps. Although subdural effusion may occur in infants with any form of meningitis, it is most commonly seen in connection with *Hemophilus influenzae* meningitis. (**Ref.** 5, pp. 66–67)

139. **(B)** Sequelae occur in approximately one-fourth of the patients who recover. There may be severe intellectual damage. Blindness, hemiplegia, paraplegia, and quadriplegia have all occurred. (**Ref.** 5, pp. 69–71)

140. **(D)** Any part of the central nervous system, the meninges, the peripheral or cranial nerves (especially the seventh) and even muscles may be affected. In terms of the prognosis, this is generally considered a benign disease, tending to involve one or more systems of the body for many years and also tending to subside spontaneously. However, recovery of peripheral or cranial nerve palsies is generally slow. (**Ref.** 5, pp. 149–151)

141. **(A)** Any part of the nervous system may be involved; total blindness may be unilateral or bilateral. The course of this disease is characterized by a series of remissions and exacerbations extending over a number of years. Kveim-Siltzbach test is negative. (**Ref.** 5, pp. 81–82)

142. **(A)** This occurs (1) because of a septic or necrotic focus in the skull or spinal canal; (2) because a foreign substance has been in-

jected into the subarachnoid space; or (3) in association with a connective tissue disorder. Usually, CSF pressure and protein are increased and sugar is normal. If severe, fluid may be purulent. (**Ref.** 5, pp. 83–84)

143. **(B)** The patient with subdural abscess is sicker, has meningeal signs, may develop focal signs, and may develop sinus thrombosis. The mortality rate is high (25% to 40%) because of failure to make an early diagnosis. (**Ref.** 5, pp. 71–72)

144. **(D)** Inflammatory processes in adjacent tissues, such as decubitus ulcers, carbuncles, or perinephric abscesses, caused the vast majority of cases. Less commonly, hematogenous metastases or perforating wounds are the source. (**Ref.** 5, pp. 73–76)

145. **(B)** Any part of the spine may be infected, but the mid-dorsal area is the most common area involved. The most common organism found is *Staphylococcus aureus* (50% to 60% of the cases). (**Ref.** 5, p. 76)

146. **(D)** Clinical findings and lumbar puncture differentiate acute spinal epidural abscess from acute multiple sclerosis; myelography differentiates chronic spinal epidural abscess from epidural tumors or chronic adhesive arachnoiditis. Andersen's disease is a myopathy; Sotas's syndrome has been considered an endocrinopathy. (**Ref.** 5, pp. 75–76)

147. **(D)** Also, suppurative lung disease may cause metastatic brain abscesses. They arise as direct extensions from infections within the cranial cavity, or from infections secondary to fracture of the skull or neurosurgical procedures, or as metastases from infection elsewhere in the body. (**Ref.** 5, p. 89)

148. **(B)** Demyelination occurs in the cerebrum, brainstem, and spinal cord. A few cases occurring in the apparent absence of an underlying disease have been reported. Most cases have been caused by JC virus; some by SV-40 strain. (**Ref.** 5, pp. 125–126)

149. **(B)** Nervous system symptoms are unusual; they may appear very early or late in the course. The exact incidence of involve-

ment of the nervous system is unknown, but it is probably less than 1%. (**Ref.** 5, pp. 118–119)

150. **(D)** The differential diagnosis included mumps and other viruses that cause a lymphocytic meningeal reaction. Oropharyngeal excretion of EB virus can also be determined. CSF protein is normal or slightly elevated; CSF sugar is normal. (**Ref.** 5, pp. 118–119)

151. **(B)** Treatment includes stopping bacterial antibiotics and cortisone, giving amphotericin B, and controlling the diabetes. The disease is usually fatal, and death is almost inevitable when the nervous system is involved. (**Ref.** 5, p. 148)

152. **(C)** Ulnar or radial nerves may also be affected. Bacilli have been found in dorsal root ganglia, spinal cord, and brain, but they do not produce any significant lesions within the CNS. (**Ref.** 5, pp. 76–78)

153. **(B)** Mental status changes occur in nearly every case. Acute purulent meningitis may be the result of infection with almost any pathogenic bacterium, but most cases are due to *Neisseria meningitidis, Hemophilus influenzae,* and *Streptococcus pneumoniae.* (**Ref.** 5, pp. 63–64)

154. **(B)** Also, the presence of Negri bodies in brain tissue is pathognomonic. Virus isolation from the saliva, throat, and CSF should be attempted, but this is rarely successful. (**Ref.** 5, p. 111)

155. **(A)** An agglutination titer of 1:64 or higher is diagnostic. This disease should be considered in all cases of lymphocytic meningitis in which the diagnosis is obscure. (**Ref.** 5, pp. 118–119)

156. **(E)** Meningitis is relatively rare. The Frei test is used less often now. Diagnosis is either by demonstrating LGV organisms in lesion or by appropriate serologic tests. Both Tetracycline and Sulfonamide drugs are effective. (**Ref.** 9, pp. 1710–1711)

157. **(C)** It can also show an increase in serum viral antibodies. When they involve the human nervous system, both group A and

group B coxsackie viruses most frequently cause so-called aseptic meningitis. (**Ref.** 5, p. 102)

158. (D) This is relatively benign. The duration of the meningeal symptoms varies from one to four weeks, with an average of three weeks. (**Ref.** 5, pp. 112–113)

159. (G) Eosinophilic intranuclear inclusions are found in oligodendroglia. It is presumed that the demyelination is due to destruction of the oligodendroglia by the virus. (**Ref.** 5, pp. 125–126)

160. (D) Convulsions were rare. The most frequent sign of disease localized to the nervous system was dysfunction of eye movements. (**Ref.** 5, pp. 129–130)

161. (H) A presumptive viral disease; it also occurs from other puncture wounds and occasionally causes encephalitis. Complications and sequelae are almost nonexistent. (**Ref.** 9, pp. 1679–1681)

162. (A) This picture is rare after smallpox vaccination. The incidence of Landry-Guillain-Barré syndrome is increased in patients with Hodgkin's disease and may also be precipitated by pregnancy and general surgery. Newer vaccines should reduce the problem of complications. (**Ref.** 5, pp. 119–121, 609–610)

163. (F) This may affect any of the nerves of the brachial plexus. In most cases of brachial neuritis, however, no common antecedent illness, immunization, or toxic exposure is found. (**Ref.** 5, p. 101; **Ref.** 9, p. 2267)

164. (E) Caused by fleas carried by rats, differentiated from disease caused by louse-borne fleas by the complement fixation test. Chloramphenicol, tetracycline, and deoxycycline are effective. (**Ref.** 5, pp. 78–79)

165. (C) Final diagnosis depends on the results of neutralization and complement fixation tests. Clinical distinction from typhus fever may be impossible. (**Ref.** 5, pp. 79–80)

166. (B) Onset of cerebral symptoms is unrelated to height of fever. Dexamethasone is deleterious in the treatment of cerebral malaria. **(Ref. 5, pp. 171–172)**

167. (C) This may be seen in poliomyelitis after the second week of infection, during the first week, pleocytosis is usually found. Previously, the main clinical differential diagnostic possibilities were acute polio and diphtheritic polyneuropathy; both are now rare in the United States. **(Ref. 5, pp. 609–610)**

168. (B) In infectious polyneuritis, the first neurologic symptom is usually weakness of the lower extremities, followed by weakness of the upper extremities and then the facial muscles. This weakness is often accompanied by paresthesias and, unlike the course of most other neuropathies, proximal muscles are sometimes affected more than distal muscles in the early phases. **(Ref. 5, pp. 609–610)**

169. (D) This occurs in Refsum's disease. In this disease, peripheral neuropathy with hypertrophied nerves is found. CSF protein may be elevated. **(Ref. 5, pp. 509–512)**

170. (D) This suggests the possibility of serum sickness. This latter condition is common after horse serum injection. It usually lasts for four to five days and should be treated with antihistamines. **(Ref. 9, pp. 1950–1951)**

171. (D) This describes herpes zoster. The diagnosis of herpes zoster is made without difficulty when the characteristic rash is present. **(Ref. 5, pp. 115–118)**

5

Diseases Due to Toxins

DIRECTIONS (Questions 172–187): Each of the questions or incomplete statements below is followed by five suggested answers or completions. Select the ONE lettered answer or completion that is BEST in each case.

172. "Crack" produces
    A. no increase in perceptual awareness
    B. CNS changes of long duration, with a low margin of safety
    C. increased heart rate, blood pressure, and capacity for muscular work
    D. anxiety without depression
    E. cardiac standstill because of direct cardiotoxicity; anaphylaxis on application to mucous membranes does not occur

173. In morphine abstinence syndrome the
    A. temperature characteristically becomes subnormal (usually 35.5–36°C)
    B. blood pressure typically decreases by 20 mm Hg or more
    C. "sleepy yen" characteristically occurs early
    D. peak is at four to five hours
    E. occurrence of convulsions is frequent

174. In the diagnosis of opiate dependence
  A. there are usually many distinctive objective findings
  B. the nalorphine test is safe and should be used early at maximum strength
  C. the nalorphine test is reliable in meperidine dependence because meperidine is equipotent with morphine
  D. naloxone should be used at once although it lacks preventive action if given before an opioid dose
  E. none of the above

175. In hypnotic dependence
  A. mid-brain centers are the most susceptible
  B. reticular-activating system neurons are the least susceptible
  C. thresholds for electrical induction of convulsions are decreased early in chronic intoxication
  D. there is an increase in the proportion of REM sleep
  E. none of the above

176. In the hypnotic abstinence syndrome
  A. postural hypotension, nausea, and vomiting occur; psychosis may occur but is transient
  B. stereotyped, self-limited illness occurs, with a peak at 8 to 10 hours
  C. convulsions, delirium, and high fever occur rarely
  D. residual damage is common
  E. none of the above

177. In alcohol dependence
  A. alcoholic tremulous syndrome is often followed by alcoholic hallucinosis, in which the hallucinations are most often auditory
  B. delirium tremens, disorientation, and agitation are just as severe as they are in alcoholic hallucinosis
  C. a small percentage of patients with acute auditory hallucinosis report that the "voices" have persisted for as long as one to two weeks
  D. delirium tremens is the most frequent type of alcohol withdrawal syndrome but, fortunately, mortality is almost nil
  E. withdrawal syndromes are associated with dehydration, not overhydration, and temperature is subnormal

178. In the diagnosis of amphetamine dependence
   A. REM sleep shows a marked decrease when the drug is withdrawn
   B. cocaine induces a clinically indistinguishable illness
   C. paranoid psychosis, usually in association with a marked organic mental syndrome, frequently occurs
   D. visual but not auditory hallucinations occur
   E. tactile but not visual hallucinations occur

179. In the diagnosis of marijuana intoxication
   A. the development of tolerance is typical and consistent
   B. the occurrence of temporary psychotic states is one of the more dangerous features of the clinical picture
   C. tachycardia, reddened conjunctivae, and impairment of recent memory and the ability to concentrate occur, along with an increase in motor performance
   D. nystagmus does not occur
   E. none of the above

180. When lead poisoning involves the brain acutely
   A. adults are affected more than twice as often as children
   B. the prognosis is quite good for life; the morbidity is now nil
   C. lead may be demonstrated in the urine but not in the blood
   D. the CSF pressure is usually normal
   E. none of the above

181. Manganese poisoning
   A. produces liver cirrhosis, and especially renal dysfunction early, in the typical case
   B. generally occurs via the GI tract
   C. is often difficult to distinguish from paralysis agitans
   D. causes changes in the basal ganglia but not in the cerebral cortex
   E. causes a clear-cut neurologic syndrome

182. In barbiturate intoxication
   A. the drugs must be discontinued promptly
   B. the reflexes are hyperactive in more than 50% of the cases
   C. residua are expected in more than 80% of the cases
   D. hemodialysis is of no significant value
   E. none of the above

183. Prolonged phenothiazine treatment may produce hyperkinesias
   A. which usually affect the upper limbs more than the lower limbs or face
   B. which, though distressing, all disappear within a few weeks at most, after withdrawal of the drug
   C. which, when studied neuropathologically, generally demonstrate specific lesions in the basal ganglia
   D. but not acute hypotensive episodes
   E. none of the above

184. Tetanus
   A. differs from strychnine poisoning in that muscles relax between spasms in the former
   B. differs from strychnine poisoning in that jaw muscles are rarely involved in the former
   C. often produces fever
   D. produces pathologic changes in the CNS
   E. produces pathologic changes in the peripheral nervous system

185. In botulism the
   A. presenting symptom is usually dysarthria
   B. toxin is destroyed by heat
   C. CSF shows a mild pleocytosis
   D. intestines are not affected
   E. bladder is not affected

186. In the treatment of botulism
   A. neostigmine is useful
   B. antibiotics are of primary importance
   C. antitoxin is useful
   D. stomach washing should not be used
   E. enemas should not be given

187. Following ingestion of methyl alcohol
   A. the pupils are constricted
   B. there is a central scotoma
   C. the peripheral fields are normal
   D. visual loss occurs in all cases
   E. dyspnea and cyanosis are rare

DIRECTIONS (Questions 188–197): The group of questions below consists of a list of lettered headings followed by a list of numbered words, phrases, or statements. For each numbered word, phrase, or statement, select the ONE lettered heading that is most closely associated with it. Each lettered heading may be selected once, more than once, or not at all.

A. Clioquinol
B. Methyl mercury
C. Clonazepam
D. Vincristine, vinblastine
E. Isoniazid
F. Hydralazine
G. Ethambutol
H. Organophosphorus compounds
I. Gold

188. SMON

189. Anti-epileptic; weight gain side effect

190. Minamata disease

191. Headaches, loss of memory, deafness, blindness, dysphagia, dysarthria

192. Usually given intravenously; sensory neuropathy with occasional painful paresthesias of the feet

193. Interferes with vitamin B_6 absorption; lower limb weakness and paresthesias

194. Interferes with vitamin B_6 absorption; causes neuropathy, and a systemic lupus erythematosus-like picture

195. Peripheral neuropathy, cranial neuropathy, confusion

196. Optic neuritis; occasional peripheral neuropathy

197. Cholinergic block causes respiratory paralysis; later, a peripheral neuropathy occurs

DIRECTIONS (Questions 198–202): The set of lettered headings below is followed by a list of numbered words or phrases. For each numbered word or phrase select

- **A.** if the item is associated with A only
- **B.** if the item is associated with B only
- **C.** if the item is associated with both A and B
- **D.** if the item is associated with neither A nor B

- **A.** Carbon monoxide
- **B.** Ethyl alcohol
- **C.** Both
- **D.** Neither

198. Recovery may be followed by basal ganglia disease, confusion, and peripheral neuropathy

199. Flushed face, dilated pupils, rapid pulse, low blood pressure, hyporeflexia; typically not preceded by headache

200. Cherry red skin color

201. Pale, wasted appearance with low ocular tension

202. Earlier, may exhibit pyramidal signs, extrapyramidal signs, "flapping tremor"

Answers and Discussion

172. **(C)** The increase in the capacity for muscular work is due to a lessened sense of fatigue. "Crack" is a CNS stimulant of short duration which increases perceptual awareness; it produces both anxiety and depression. Treatment of an overdose is symptomatic, with respiratory and cardiovascular monitoring, along with support systems. (**Ref.** 5, p. 911)

173. **(C)** The morphine abstinence syndrome is stereotyped, self-limited and not dangerous to life in the absence of serious physical disease. With morphine and heroin, withdrawal symptoms peak at 36 to 48 hours and most symptoms subside over the next 5 to 10 days. Convulsions or cardiovascular collapse are rare. (**Ref.** 9, p. 57)

174. **(E)** Diagnosis is usually made by the history and confirmed by withholding drugs, thereby allowing signs of abstinence to appear. The abstinence syndrome may be precipitated within minutes in opiate-dependent persons by administration of a narcotic antagonist, although there are no medical indications for this diagnostic procedure. (**Ref.** 9, pp. 56–57)

175. **(E)** Hypnotics raise the threshold of excitation of all types of neurons and depress all kinds of central reflexes. Both drug disposition and pharmacodynamic tolerance of the depressants develop rapidly with repeated administration. REM sleep is reduced. (**Ref.** 9, pp. 52–54)

176. (E) In contrast with opiate abstinence, hypnotic abstinence is dangerous to life. The first manifestation of this syndrome might be considered the rebound increase in nightly REM sleep, associated nightmares, and a sense of having slept badly (after barbiturate or benzodiazepine discontinuance). Some symptoms may last weeks or months. (**Ref.** 9, pp. 53–54)

177. (A) Several tremulous, convulsive, delerious, and other states occur after cessation or reduction in alcohol intake; although described separately, they are variants of the same basic disorder. In delerium tremens, hallucinations are most commonly visual. Temperature is usually elevated. Untreated patients have approximately a 15% mortality. (**Ref.** 9, pp. 50–51)

178. (B) Diagnosis is usually made by the history and especially if the patient presents with a paranoid psychosis that clears in a few days after a period of sleep. After the drug's effects have worn off, affected individuals have a lower threshold for precipitation of psychotic episodes, even after long, intervening periods. (**Ref.** 9, pp. 53–55)

179. (B) The history is most important; also suggestive is a rapidly clearing schizophreniform episode. The most common adverse effects are simple depression, acute panic reactions, and paranoid ideation. Motor performance decreases; nystagmus and ataxia have been noted. (**Ref.** 9, pp. 57–58)

180. (E) Treatment with BAL, calcium, EDTA, and other substances has reduced mortality greatly; it has reduced morbidity somewhat. Common residua include dementia, seizures, ataxia, and spasticity. CSF may show marked increase in pressure. Lead is found in both blood and urine. (**Ref.** 5, p. 921)

181. (C) A middle-aged patient who is unknowingly exposed (usually by inhalation) to this toxin and then develops a Parkinsonian syndrome presents a problem in differential diagnosis. Rigidity and hypokinesia can be improved by the use of L-dopa. (**Ref.** 5, p. 924; **Ref.** 9, p. 2392)

182. (E) Even after being in a coma for a week, patients who recover usually have no residua. Hemodialysis can help some patients in prolonged, severe coma and those who have ingested lethal doses. (**Ref.** 5, pp. 911–912)

183. (E) The Parkinson-like syndrome disappears on drug withdrawal; the dystonic or choreic movements may persist. If dyskinetic or akathitic symptoms are too distressing, treatment with dopamine-depleting drugs may help; reserpine is preferred by some investigators. (**Ref.** 5, pp. 674–676; **Ref.** 9, p. 2094)

184. (C) The history of the wound is helpful. The mortality rate is still high (over 50%). There are no pathologic changes in either the CNS or the peripheral nervous system. (**Ref.** 5, pp. 176–178)

185. (B) Constipation and urinary retention occur. Bulbar involvement due to polio is excluded by the normal CSF. Myasthenia gravis shows a different EMG response. (**Ref.** 5, pp. 178–179)

186. (C) Bivalent antitoxin is used for poisoning by meat or vegetable; type E (trivalent) should be used if fish poisoning is suspected. A respirator may also be needed. The stomach should be washed. (**Ref.** 5, pp. 178–179)

187. (B) Visual loss is the only neurologic sequela in those who recover. Peripheral fields are constricted and the pupils may be large. Treatment includes gastric lavage, administration of alkali, and hemodialysis. (**Ref.** 5, pp. 925–926)

188. (A) Loss of vision, ascending numbness, motor weakness, and autonomic dysfunction are found. This is similar to Jamaican neuropathy. (**Ref.** 5, p. 696)

189. (C) Atypical absence and myoclonus attacks. (**Ref.** 5, pp. 798, 802)

190. (B) This is found in antifungal agents (grain), as well as in tuna and swordfish. Symptoms may develop weeks or months after ingestion. (**Ref.** 5, pp. 924–925)

191. (B) Fatigue and apathy; residua are often severe. The fetus is especially vulnerable. (**Ref.** 5, pp. 924–925)

192. (D) Used in lymphomas and leukemias. Neurotoxicity is well known with vincristine but rare with vinblastine; however, the latter is highly toxic to bone marrow. **(Ref. 9, pp. 1125–1126)**

193. (E) Can be prevented by giving pyridoxine. In adults, isoniazid produces neuritis and diarrhea. In children, it causes anemia and convulsions. **(Ref. 9, pp. 1233–1234)**

194. (F) Psychoses and tremors have also been reported. The many drugs able to induce features of systemic lupus erythematosus do not share common structural or chemical properties. **(Ref. 9, p. 103)**

195. (I) Sodium aurothiomalate is used in rheumatoid arthritis. Most prominent side effects, however, involve bone marrow, kidney, and skin. **(Ref. 9, p. 2003)**

196. (G) Confusion has also been reported, along with possible hallucinations. The optic neuropathy is usually reversible if the drug is discontinued promptly. **(Ref. 9, p. 1687)**

197. (H) Tri-ortho-cresyl phosphate has caused the largest number of cases of human neuropathy. Patients who do not become comatose usually recover, without permanent sequelae. **(Ref. 5, p. 926)**

198. (A) There may be loss of memory and signs of focal brain damage. Patients who do not become comatose usually recover, with permanent sequelae. **(Ref. 9, p. 2369)**

199. (B) At a blood level of 150 mg%, acute intoxication is likely; over 250 mg%, coma occurs; 400 to 500 mg% often leads to death. Death is due to respiratory depression; therefore, artificial ventilation in an intensive care unit is the mainstay of treatment. **(Ref. 5, pp. 899–900)**

200. (A) In doubtful cases, spectroscopic blood examination is performed. Patients with neurologic abnormalities should be considered for treatment with hyperbaric oxygen even if carboxyhemoglobin levels are low. **(Ref. 9, p. 2369)**

201. **(D)** This is found in diabetes mellitus. In diabetic coma, one checks for odor of acetone on the breath and the presence of sugar in the urine. **(Ref.** 5, p. 21)

202. **(D)** This suggests liver disease. Asterixis occurs bilaterally in metabolic encephalopathy; unilaterally, it suggests structural brain disease. **(Ref.** 9, p. 2065)

6

Metabolic Diseases

DIRECTIONS (Questions 203–241): Each of the questions or incomplete statements below is followed by suggested answers or completions. Select the ONE that is BEST in each case.

203. In polyneuropathy, the pathologic process does not
   A. result in a mild reduction in motor conduction velocities in nerve fiber degenerative neuropathies
   B. result in a marked reduction in motor conduction velocities in nerve fiber demyelinating neuropathies
   C. involve nerve fiber degeneration primarily in ischemic situations
   D. involve segmental demyelination predominantly in diabetes
   E. none of the above

204. In beriberi
   A. myocardial disease does not occur
   B. polyneuritis does not occur
   C. the blood pyruvate level is decreased; thiamine is administered
   D. A and B but not C
   E. none of the above

205. Refsum's syndrome does not include
   A. a chronic motor and sensory polyneuropathy
   B. retinitis pigmentosa
   C. deafness and cerebellar ataxia
   D. peripheral nerve thickening caused by excessive collagen
   E. none of the above

206. The cranial nerve most often involved in polyneuritis is the
   A. fifth
   B. seventh
   C. ninth
   D. tenth
   E. twelfth

207. The treatment of choice for subacute combined degeneration is
   A. oral folic acid
   B. oral vitamin B_{12}
   C. parenteral folic acid
   D. parenteral vitamin B_{12}
   E. none of the above

208. Hypophysectomy has been reported to help
   A. limit the development of the rete mirabile in moyamoya disease
   B. in the retinal vascular changes of diabetics
   C. in the proliferative retinal changes of diabetics
   D. in the subhyaloid hemorrhages of diabetes
   E. none of the above

209. Sickle cell anemia
   A. does not cause subarachnoid hemorrhage
   B. can produce neurologic manifestations independent, temporally, of the crises
   C. does not cause subdural hemorrhage
   D. causes extension of marrow through the inner skull table and therefore a "hair-on-end" appearance
   E. symptoms afflict a large percentage of individuals whose blood shows the typical anomaly

210. Most frequently reported with the use of contraceptive hormones are
- **A.** temporal lobe phenomena
- **B.** migraine and monocular diplopia
- **C.** atypical facial pain
- **D.** neuro-ocular disorders
- **E.** dyskinesias, generally transient

211. In adult myxedema
- **A.** slow speech occurs
- **B.** peripheral neuropathy and myopathy are rare
- **C.** myotonia does not occur
- **D.** delirium is frequent
- **E.** sudden coma is not uncommon

212. In adult myxedema
- **A.** the CSF protein is normal
- **B.** Kocher-Debre-Semelaigne syndrome is frequent
- **C.** absence of alpha waves in the EEG has been reported
- **D.** some laboratory abnormalities can be demonstrated even after adequate therapy
- **E.** a low basal metabolic rate alone can make the diagnosis

213. In hyperthyroidism
- **A.** psychosis occurs
- **B.** infrequent winking occurs, but not impaired convergence
- **C.** paresis of the trunk and extremities is found, but not familial periodic paralysis
- **D.** weakness is greatly increased by small doses of curare
- **E.** when myasthenia gravis is associated, the former almost invariably precedes the latter

214. In the differential diagnosis of neurologic dysfunction with thyrotoxicosis, myasthenia gravis may not generally be excluded by
- **A.** the neostigmine test
- **B.** the curare test
- **C.** any known test
- **D.** the edrophonium test
- **E.** none of the above

215. The findings in hypoparathyroidism include
    A. calcification in the basal ganglia
    B. sensory but not motor features
    C. seizures, usually psychomotor
    D. choked discs frequently
    E. chorea but not torticollis

216. In pseudohypoparathyroidism
    A. convulsions occur
    B. the parathyroids are hypoplastic
    C. calcium and phosphorus are normal in one form of this illness yet tetany still occurs
    D. the stature is characteristically lengthened, the face angular
    E. none of the above

217. In hyperparathyroidism
    A. the neurologic onset may be marked by back pain
    B. psychosis does not occur
    C. plain roentgenograms are of little value
    D. polyuria and polydipsia are uncommon
    E. vertebral cyst formation not uncommonly is a cause of spinal cord compression

218. Hypoglycemia
    A. occurs in hepatic and pituitary but not adrenal damage
    B. produces myoclonic jerks in infancy related to a deficiency of leucine
    C. causes autonomic activity lasting for hours
    D. is usually due to islet cell tumor of the head of the pancreas
    E. produces no demonstrable cerebral damage

219. The findings in hypoglycemia
    A. do not include diplopia and nystagmus
    B. do not include aphasia
    C. do not include hemiparesis
    D. include grand mal but not Jacksonian seizure
    E. none of the above

220. Dwarfism is
    A. found in suprasellar tumors
    B. associated with mental retardation in hypopituitarism

    C. associated with macrogenitalia in hypopituitarism
    D. associated with Pott's disease but not celiac disease
    E. associated with achondroplasia but not pancreatic insufficiency

221. Diabetes insipidus
    A. is much more likely to be primary than secondary
    B. is more likely to occur in a case of hypothalamic tumor than in a case of xanthomatosis
    C. causes a significant increase in specific gravity of the urine when fluids are withheld for 12 hours
    D. usually produces an impairment in general health
    E. none of the above

222. Leukemia
    A. produces cranial neuropathy, especially of the abducens; rarely, spinal neuropathies occur
    B. produces paraplegia
    C. produces no change in CSF pressure or protein
    D. is complicated by progressive multifocal leukoencephalopathy in a large percentage of cases
    E. frequently causes hemiplegia and aphasia

223. Paget's disease
    A. produces platybasia early
    B. most often produces blindness
    C. infrequently causes facial palsy
    D. usually causes disability only when the skull or spine is involved
    E. seldom causes deafness

224. Leontiasis ossea
    A. frequently includes a familial tendency
    B. is first noted clinically in the fourth to sixth decades
    C. produces exophthalmos, optic atrophy, and other cranial neuropathies
    D. has a distinct racial preference
    E. none of the above

225. In Graves' disease, associated neurologic syndromes include
    A. myasthenia gravis and familial periodic paralysis
    B. exophthalmic ophthalmoplegia and dermatomyositis
    C. chronic thyrotoxic myopathy and polyarteritis
    D. familial periodic paralysis and polymyalgia rheumatica
    E. none of the above

226. Myxedema
    A. has been reported with myasthenia gravis in many patients
    B. not infrequently produces myoedema but not myotonia
    C. may include the Kocher-Debre-Semelaigne syndrome
    D. very frequently causes cranial neuropathies
    E. none of the above

227. In myxedema
    A. carpal tunnel syndrome occurs rarely
    B. polyneuritis is found in approximately 90% of the cases
    C. cranial neuropathies and psychoses are noted frequently
    D. infant Hercules syndrome occurs frequently
    E. none of the above

228. Acute porphyria
    A. commonly produces abdominal pain and gastric dilatation
    B. commonly produces cloudy urine
    C. usually causes widespread areas of necrosis in the CNS
    D. commonly causes convulsions
    E. causes weakness, which is typically most prominent proximally

229. In thyrotoxic myopathy, the
    A. electromyogram shows fibrillation potentials
    B. weakness usually occurs when other thyrotoxic signs are less prominent
    C. reflexes are diminished
    D. distal weakness is prominent
    E. iliopsoas is particularly involved

230. In hereditary sensory neuropathy
    A. proprioception is preserved
    B. perforating ulcers occur
    C. thermal sensibility is preserved

D. sensory deficits are first noted in the third to fourth decades
E. reflexes are normal

231. The neurologic findings of acute porphyria include
   A. dysarthria
   B. frequently, both facial diplegia and cutaneous sensory loss
   C. amblyopia
   D. normal tendon reflexes
   E. extremity weakness, usually most marked proximally

232. The convulsive seizures of hypoparathyroidism
   A. are usually Jacksonian
   B. do not usually respond to anticonvulsants
   C. are not usually associated with signs of tetany
   D. occur infrequently
   E. are not accompanied by psychotic manifestations

233. The neurologic abnormalities in hypoparathyroidism do not include
   A. calcifications in the basal ganglia
   B. choked discs
   C. bursts of 2–5/sec waves on the EEG
   D. elevated CSF protein
   E. lowered threshold of electrical excitability of the nerve

234. Precocious puberty in males has been reported with
   A. hypoplasia of the adrenal cortex
   B. hamartomas of the hypothalamus
   C. no other tumors of the hypothalamus
   D. decreased excretion of 17-ketosteroids
   E. its equally common counterpart, feminization of males due to estrogen-producing tumors

235. In Hodgkin's disease of the nervous system, the
   A. brain is usually invaded
   B. spinal cord is usually invaded
   C. brain is usually involved more than the spinal cord
   D. meninges are usually invaded
   E. cauda equina is usually invaded

236. The pathogenesis of thrombotic thrombocytopenic purpura includes
   A. occlusion of arteries, arterioles, and capillaries, and hemolytic anemia
   B. sparing of vessels supplying the heart
   C. noninvolvement of renal vessels
   D. thrombocytopenia persisting between attacks
   E. none of the above

237. Treatment of leukemic involvement of the CNS does not include
   A. steroids
   B. 6-mercaptopurine
   C. x-ray therapy to the entire skull and spine
   D. methotrexate
   E. BCNU, CCNU

238. In the Guillain-Barré syndrome
   A. the cell count is usually elevated, the protein normal
   B. the albuminocytologic dissociation is pathognomonic
   C. facial diplegia is uncommon
   D. the clinical picture usually includes prominent sensory changes
   E. none of the above

239. Cervical radiculomyelopathy associated with spondylosis
   A. uncommonly causes pain in the upper extremities and neck
   B. commonly causes sphincteric disturbances
   C. can be diagnosed by myelography
   D. commonly causes overt sensory loss
   E. none of the above

240. In the neurologic disorders associated with diabetes
   A. the pathologic findings are restricted to the peripheral nerves
   B. ocular palsies do not occur bilaterally
   C. posterior myelopathy and orthostatic hypotension do not occur
   D. Charcot joint does not occur
   E. none of the above

241. Adrenal cortex tumors may produce
   A. attacks of recurrent weakness simulating familial periodic paralysis
   B. hypertension with hypokalemia, hyponatremia, and alkalosis
   C. hypertension with hyponatremia but without hypokalemia
   D. hypertension with hypokalemia and acidosis
   E. none of the above

DIRECTIONS (Questions 242–245): The group of questions below consists of a list of lettered headings followed by a list of numbered words, phrases, or statements. For each numbered word, phrase, or statement, select the ONE lettered heading that is most closely associated with it. Each lettered heading may be selected once, more than once, or not at all.

Questions 242–245:

   A. Morquio's syndrome
   B. Hunter's syndrome
   C. Scheie's syndrome
   D. Hurler's syndrome
   E. Sanfilippo's syndrome

242. Aortic regurgitation reported, along with pigmentary degeneration of retina, carpal tunnel syndrome; normal intelligence

243. Clouding of cornea reported, along with cervical cord compression due to atlantoaxial subluxation; normal intelligence

244. Patients with the mild form may be asymptomatic

245. Prominent mental involvement; seizures

DIRECTIONS (Questions 246–250): The set of lettered headings below is followed by a list of numbered words or phrases. For each numbered word or phrase select
   A. if the item is associated with A only
   B. if the item is associated with B only
   C. if the item is associated with both A and B
   D. if the item is associated with neither A nor B

Questions 246–250:

   A. Maple syrup urine disease
   B. Hartnup disease
   C. Both
   D. Neither

246. Defective amino acid transport into small intestine cells and proximal renal tubules

247. Convulsions, decerebrate rigidity, and coma

248. Involves leucine, isoleucine, and valine

249. No treatment helps

250. Inborn metabolic error

DIRECTIONS (Questions 251–255): The group of questions below consists of lettered headings followed by a list of numbered words or statements. For each numbered word or statement, select the ONE lettered heading that is most closely associated with it. Each lettered heading may be selected once, more than once, or not at all.

Questions 251–255:

   A. Peripheral neuropathy, cerebellar degeneration, and pigmentary retinopathy
   B. Retinal hemorrhage and occasional cerebral hemorrhage
   C. Night blindness

D. Polyneuropathy, spastic ataxia, pellagra, and psychosis-dementia

E. Peripheral neuropathy, Wernicke-Korsakoff syndrome

251. Vitamin A deficiency

252. Vitamin C deficiency

253. Vitamin E deficiency

254. Nicotinic acid deficiency

255. Thiamine deficiency

Answers and Discussion

203. (E) In chronic neuropathies there is also evidence of partial nerve regeneration. After axonal degeneration, regeneration is slow and incomplete. After demyelination, recovery, if it occurs, is rapid and more complete. (**Ref.** 4, pp. 417, 419)

204. (E) In the tropics, this is usually due to dietary deficiency; in temperate climates, to defective absorption. The latter is caused by some forms of GI disease of alcoholism. (**Ref.** 4, p. 494)

205. (E) This is inherited via a recessive gene, with a resultant defect in lipid metabolism. The defect may be circumvented by a diet that excludes phytanic acid. (**Ref.** 4, p. 421)

206. (B) Sometimes ophthalmoplegia or bulbar paralysis occurs. In Landry-Guillain-Barré syndrome, even the optic nerves may be involved (papilledema), and eighth nerve dysfunction may cause deafness. (**Ref.** 4, pp. 421–422)

207. (D) Administration of folic acid alone may cause a neurologic crisis because of the sudden uptake by the marrow, for erythropoiesis, of the little available vitamin B_{12}. Parenteral vitamin B_{12} must be continued for life. (**Ref.** 4, p. 499)

208. (B) Hypophysectomy is of no value in diabetic vitreous scarring, glaucoma, and cataracts. Furthermore, with the advent of photocoagulation, the use of hypophysectomy for proliferative retinopathy has been largely abandoned. (**Ref.** 9, p. 1378)

209. (B) The production of ischemia and hemorrhagic lesions in the nervous system, plus thromboses and infarction in bones and viscera, results in a variety of clinical manifestations. Neurologic complications also include bacterial meningitis, subarachnoid hemorrhage, and subdural hemorrhage. (**Ref.** 5, pp. 844–845)

210. (D) The main side effects appear to be vascular, namely, hypertension, migraine, and cerebrovascular lesions. However, because of the many patients taking these hormones and the occasional occurrence of all of these conditions in women of the age groups concerned, it is difficult to assess the role of the hormone with regard to these conditions. (**Ref.** 5, pp. 227–228)

211. (A) Diffuse involvement of the CNS, as well as the peripheral nervous system and muscles, may occur. Although sudden coma is rare, if untreated it has a high mortality rate. (**Ref.** 5, pp. 829–830)

212. (C) CSF protein is increased. All laboratory values become normal with adequate treatment. Treatment of myxedema is 12.5–25 mg levothyroxine, with a gradual increase if needed and if tolerated. Kocher-Debre-Semelaigne syndrome occurs in children with generalized enlargement, or hypertrophy, of muscles. (**Ref.** 5, pp. 829–830)

213. (A) Neurologic symptoms are commonly limited to abnormalities in mental status and in ocular and motor systems. Oropharyngeal weakness or ophthalmoparesis almost always indicates myasthenia. Myasthenia gravis may precede or follow thyrotoxicosis but, most often, the two diseases occur simultaneously. (**Ref.** 5, pp. 831–832)

214. (E) Patients may have both diseases simultaneously and are then given a combination of therapies. About 5% of patients with myasthenia gravis have hyperthyroidism. (**Ref.** 5, pp. 831–832)

215. (A) Tetany is common; convulsions are often resistant to anticonvulsants. Various dyskinesias have been reported. Tetany may be manifested by carpopedal spasm; latent tetany may be demonstrated by the Chvostek sign, Trousseau sign, and Erb sign. Papilledema has been reported in a few cases only. (**Ref.** 5, pp. 832–833)

216. (A) Administration of parathyroid hormone does not increase phosphate excretion or serum calcium; normal values of calcium and phosphorus occur in pseudo-pseudohypoparathyroidism (and tetany is absent). This probably represents a forme fruste of pseudohypoparathyroidism. The parathyroids are histologically normal or hyperplastic. (**Ref.** 5, pp. 832–833)

217. (A) Early neurologic complaints usually include pains and weakness but mental changes may occur; plain x-ray findings including "ground glass" calvarium are characteristic. There may be mild to moderate muscle atrophy. Coma may occur. Vertebral cyst formation is a rare cause of spinal cord or root compression. (**Ref.** 5, pp. 834–836)

218. (C) Most instances of spontaneous hypoglycemia are said to be due to one of three conditions: functional hypoglycemia, hyperinsulinism with demonstrable pancreatic lesions, or organic liver disease. Hypoglycemia may occur with islet cell tumors or may be associated with functional overactivity of the cells. It also occurs with severe damage to the pituitary or the adrenal. The brain may show degenerative changes. (**Ref.** 5, pp. 836–838)

219. (E) The neurologic examination is usually normal, except during the actual hypoglycemic episode; sympathetic disturbances usually precede disturbances of the CNS. However, amyotrophy as a result of damage to ventral horn cells has been reported. A variety of seizures may occur. (**Ref.** 5, pp. 836–838)

220. (A) The exact role of the pituitary in this disorder is unknown; sexual development is usually subnormal. Occasionally, however, sexual development is normal and the dwarf is able to produce offspring (eg, Barnum and Bailey's famous dwarf, Tom Thumb). In pituitary dwarfism, mental status is normal. (**Ref.** 5, p. 824)

221. (E) This is a relatively rare disorder whether primary or secondary; failure to concentrate the urine when fluids are withheld differentiates it from hysterical polydipsia. The investigation of diabetes insipidus includes special attention to visual acuity and visual fields, along with skull x-rays and CT or MRI. Secondary diabetes insipidus is an important symptom of hypothalamic disease. (**Ref. 5**, pp. 824–826)

222. **(B)** Foci occur in cranial or peripheral nerves, epidural space, meninges, and CNS parenchyma, but probably most often in the seventh cranial nerve. Focal signs of cerebral damage are infrequent, except for hypothalamic syndromes such as diabetes insipidus. The CSF pressure and protein are increased, with infiltration of the meninges. (**Ref. 5**, pp. 851–852)

223. **(D)** The neurologic defects are usually due to bony overgrowth pressing on the CNS or nerve roots. Skull x-rays show an enormous skull with a "cotton wool" appearance of the bones of the vault. Deafness is more common than unilateral facial palsy. (**Ref. 5**, pp. 863–866)

224. **(C)** Monostotic and polyostotic forms of fibrous dysplasia occur; the polyostotic form includes endocrine dysfunction as one of its features. In addition, café au lait spots and femur involvement occur in the latter. There is no racial nor sexual preference and the family history is negative. (**Ref. 5**, p. 866)

225. **(A)** In a combination of Graves' disease and myasthenia gravis, both diseases are treated; in a combination of Graves' disease and familial periodic paralysis, treatment is directed to Graves' disease. Patients with thyrotoxic periodic paralysis are susceptible to spontaneous or induced attacks during the period of hyperthyroidism; when the patients become euthyroid, spontaneous attacks cease. Graves' disease also has been associated with chronic thyrotoxic myopathy and with exophthalmic ophthalmoplegia. (**Ref. 5**, pp. 723, 831–832)

226. **(C)** The CNS peripheral nervous system and muscular systems may all be involved. Dysarthria or hoarseness are probably related to myxedematous infiltration of the tongue and palate rather than to twelfth or tenth cranial neuropathies. Association with myasthenia gravis has occurred in a few patients. Cranial neuropathies occur relatively infrequently. (**Ref. 5**, pp. 829–831)

227. **(E)** All occur, but infrequently except for carpal tunnel syndrome (frequent) and almost half of the patients report pains and paresthesias. The polyneuropathy clears rapidly with thyroid replacement therapy. (**Ref. 5**, pp. 615, 829–831)

228. **(A)** This typically includes GI, neurologic, and psychiatric symptoms and signs. GI symptoms are attributed to autonomic neuropathy. Other autonomic abnormalities include hypertension and tachycardia. Urine may be bright red. Even in fatal cases it may be difficult to demonstrate any histologic lesions. (**Ref. 5**, pp. 544–546)

229. **(E)** There are no fibrillation potentials on the EMG but gross muscular twitchings may be seen. Weakness and wasting are greatest in the muscles of the pelvic girdle, especially the iliopsoas and, to a lesser extent, in the muscles of the shoulder girdle. Reflexes are normal or hyperactive. (**Ref. 5**, pp. 831–832)

230. **(B)** This group includes dominantly inherited or type I; an autosomal recessive form that resembles type I; congenital sensory neuropathy with anhydrosis; hereditary sensory neuropathy with spastic paraparesis and familial dysautonomia. Proprioception, thermal sensibility, pain, light touch, and reflexes are all lost. (**Ref. 5**, p. 606)

231. **(C)** Any of the cranial nerves may be involved. Primarily, motor polyneuropathy may progress rapidly to flaccid quadriplegia, respiratory and bulbar paralysis, and ophthalmoplegia. (**Ref. 5**, pp. 544–546, 606–607)

232. **(B)** These are usually grand mal but may be bizarre, leading to the erroneous diagnosis of hysteria. They tend to occur frequently and respond poorly to anticonvulsants. Tetany is present in practically all patients with hypoparathyroidism. (**Ref. 5**, pp. 832–833)

233. **(D)** The basal ganglia calcifications do not, however, apparently correlate with the variety of dyskinesias reported in these conditions. These include chorea, torticollis, athetosis, dystonia, paralysis agitans, oculogyric crises, and other basal ganglia symptoms. (**Ref. 5**, p. 833)

234. (B) Other hypothalamic tumors can produce this, also. In the female before puberty, adrenal androgenic hyperplasia causes virilism. Virilism after the age of puberty is not uncommon. In these instances, there is increased excretion of urinary keto-steroids. (**Ref.** 5, p. 839)

235. (D) The granulomatous masses invade the meninges; the spinal cord is affected primarily by compression or by occlusion of its blood supply. Sometimes there is collapse of affected vertebrae. Invasion of brain or cord is rare. (**Ref.** 5, pp. 847–851)

236. (A) In a few cases, pathologic features have suggested a relationship with collagen disease. Diagnosis is based upon the triad of microangiopathic hemolytic anemia, thrombocytopenia, and cerebral symptoms and signs. It is noteworthy that thrombotic thrombocytopenic purpura-like syndrome can occur in patients with malignancies following chemotherapy. Hyaline thrombi occlude arterioles and capillaries of virtually every tissue. (**Ref.** 9, p. 1052)

237. (E) Intrathecal methotrexate or aminopterin is used because meningeal leukemia intervenes so frequently while there is systemic (bone marrow) remission, it has become standard practice to follow induction therapy with prophylactic treatment of the CNS. (**Ref.** 5, pp. 851–852)

238. (E) A similar syndrome occurs in polyneuritis of various causes. One looks for a combination of a history of subacute development of symmetric motor or sensorimotor neuropathy following viral illness, immunization, or surgery, together with electrophysiologic findings consistent with segmental demyelination, along with an elevated CSF protein content and a normal CSF cell count. (**Ref.** 5, pp. 609–612)

239. (C) The roots are damaged by narrowing of the foramina, the cord, by compression, and perhaps by other factors, including circulatory conditions. In cervical spondylotic myelopathy, the most common symptom is spastic gait disorder. Weakness and wasting of the hands may be seen. (**Ref.** 5, pp. 409–411)

240. (E) Pathologic changes in "diabetic polyneuritis" have been found in peripheral nerves, nerve roots, posterior columns of the spinal cord, and ventral horn cells. Diabetes mellitus is the most frequent cause of neuropathy in the United States. Three types occur: symmetric distal polyneuropathy, autonomic neuropathy, and mononeuropathy or mononeuropathy multiples. (**Ref.** 5, pp. 614–615)

241. (A) Tetany may also occur. Primary aldosteronism, due to a tumor of the adrenal cortex, also produces hypertension, polyuria, alkalosis, hypernatremia, and hyperkalemia. (**Ref.** 5, pp. 839–840)

242. (C) The life span may be normal, depending on the cardiac course. (**Ref.** 5, pp. 516–523)

243. (A) Keratosulfate is found in Morquio's syndrome. In this group, screening tests may be falsely negative, especially in the Sanfilippo and Morquio syndromes. (**Ref.** 5, pp. 518–519)

244. (B) This is an X-linked recessive syndrome. This refers to the type of Hunter's syndrome in which patients may be asymptomatic. Another type of Hunter's syndrome is a severe form. (**Ref.** 5, p. 518)

245. (E) Excess heparitin sulfate occurs. These patients deteriorate neurologically, with progressive dementia, spastic quadriparesis, tetraballism, athetosis, incontinence, and seizures. (**Ref.** 5, p. 518)

246. (B) Impaired absorption of tryptophan. This is associated with intermittent cerebellar ataxia and a photosensitive rash. (**Ref.** 5, pp. 497–498)

247. (A) Rapid course in early infancy. Some patients have presented with pseudotumor cerebri or with fluctuating ophthalmoplegia. (**Ref.** 5, pp. 493–496)

248. (A) Accumulation of keto acids in the urine causes the maple syrup odor. The condition is diagnosed by the characteristic odor of the patient and by a positive 2,4-dinitrophenylhydrazine test on the urine. (**Ref.** 5, pp. 493–496)

249. (D) Maple syrup disease helped by synthetic diet low in branched-chain amino acids; Hartnup disease by nicotinamide. However, the tendency for symptoms to remit spontaneously and for general improvement to occur with improved dietary intake and advancing age make such therapy for Hartnup disease difficult to evaluate. (**Ref.** 5, pp. 493–498)

250. (C) With genetic disorders, it is important to begin treatment early. See the caveat (in the preceding answer) regarding treatment evaluation of Hartnup disease. In maple syrup disease, as a consequence of dietary therapy, the reduced white matter density demonstrable on CT scan reverts to normal. (**Ref.** 5, pp. 493–498)

251. (C) This may also produce pseudotumor in children. (**Ref.** 9, p. 2138)

252. (B) This may also produce occasional cerebral hemorrhage. (**Ref.** 9, p. 2138)

253. (A) This may also produce ophthalmoplegia. (**Ref.** 9, pp. 2138, 2140)

254. (D) This may also produce amblyopia. (**Ref.** 9, p. 2138)

255. (E) This may also produce amblyopia, cerebellar degeneration, cerebral atrophy. (**Ref.** 9, p. 2138)

7

Anomalies

DIRECTIONS (Questions 256–259): Each of the questions or incomplete statements below is followed by suggested answers or completions. Select the ONE that is BEST in each case.

256. Platybasia clinically may not simulate
  A. multiple sclerosis
  B. syringomyelia
  C. posterior fossa tumor
  D. Arnold-Chiari malformation
  E. none of the above

257. Spina bifida is associated with defective development of the
  A. spinal cord or brain stem
  B. cerebellum but not cerebrum
  C. cerebrum but not cerebellum
  D. spinal cord but not brain stem
  E. brain stem but not spinal cord

258. In the Arnold-Chiari malformation
  A.   symptoms and signs of injury to the cerebellum, medulla, and cranial nerves occur
  B.   the picture may simulate that of posterior fossa tumor but not that of multiple sclerosis
  C.   the picture may simulate that of syringomyelia but not that of platybasia
  D.   symptoms are most often delayed until adult life
  E.   hydrocephalus is uncommon

259. The symptoms associated with a cervical rib
  A.   are more common in males
  B.   frequently include Horner's syndrome
  C.   are more motor than sensory
  D.   begin with pain most often
  E.   none of the above

DIRECTIONS (Questions 260–265): The group of questions below consists of a list of lettered headings followed by a list of numbered words, phrases, or statements. For each numbered word, phrase, or statement, select the ONE lettered heading that is most closely associated with it. Each lettered heading may be selected once, more than once, or not at all.

Questions 260–265:

  A.   Arnold-Chiari malformation
  B.   Basilar impression
  C.   Fusion of cervical vertebrae (Klippel-Feil syndrome)
  D.   18 trisomy syndrome, 13 trisomy syndrome

260. The odontoid process is above Chamberlain's line

261. "Mirror movements" of the upper extremities

262. Occiput and cervical spine are displaced

263. Facial deformities, flexion abnormalities of fingers

264. Seldom causes neurologic symptoms unless other lesions are associated

265. Primarily a defect of neural tissue; hydrocephalus usually present; symptoms may begin in adult life

---

DIRECTIONS (Questions 266–270): The set of lettered headings below is followed by a list of numbered words or phrases. For each numbered word or phrase select

    A. if the item is associated with A only
    B. if the item is associated with B only
    C. if the item is associated with both A and B
    D. if the item is associated with neither A nor B

Questions 266–270:

    A. Apert's syndrome
    B. Crouzon's syndrome
    C. Both
    D. Neither

266. Tower skull

267. Exophthalmos

268. "Parrot-beak" nose

269. Premature closure of lambdoid sutures alone

270. Syndactyly of hands and feet

Answers and Discussion

256. (E) The great variation possible in the clinical picture is due to variation in the degree of compression of the brain stem, cerebellum, and cervical cord plus the stretching of cranial nerves. "Platybasia," "basilar impression," and "basilar invagination" are terms that some writers use interchangeably for the skeletal malformation in which the base of the skull is flattened on the cervical spine. (**Ref.** 5, p. 483)

257. (A) It may also be associated with meningoceles, meningomyeloceles, congenital tumors, hydrocephalus, or developmental defects in other parts of the body. Spina bifida occulta may be present without any neurologic symptoms. (**Ref.** 5, pp. 475–478)

258. (A) In the adult, the diagnosis should be considered when involvement of the cerebellum, medulla, and lower cranial nerves occur in a patient with spina bifida. The diagnosis can be established by myelography, CT, or MRI. The adult form may simulate posterior fossa tumor, multiple sclerosis, or syrinx. (**Ref.** 5, pp. 480–482)

259. (D) The ribs are frequently bilateral but the symptoms are usually unilateral. It must be remembered that a cervical rib is a congenital abnormality that may be present in cases of syringomyelia; its presence alone is therefore not proof that the rib is the cause of the symptoms. Most patients are women and symptoms are more sensory than motor. (**Ref.** 4, p. 407)

260. **(B)** There is distortion of the stem and cranial nerves. The term "basilar impression" specifically is applied to an upward displacement of the occipital bone and cervical spine, with protrusion of the odontoid process into the foramen magnum. (**Ref. 5,** p. 483)

261. **(C)** This condition is present from birth, decreasing with increasing age. In this phenomenon, voluntary movements of one arm are involuntarily imitated to a greater or lesser degree by the other. (**Ref. 5,** pp. 484–485)

262. **(B)** Minor degrees of platybasia basilar invagination may cause no symptoms. Basilar impression is rare. Neurologic symptoms, when present, usually develop in childhood or early in adult life. (**Ref.** 5, p. 483)

263. **(D)** Multisystemic defects are found in both syndromes. Mental retardation, growth failure, and multiple congenital defects should arouse suspicion of a chromosome aberration. (**Ref.** 9, p. 167)

264. **(C)** Syrinx, defects of the cord, brain stem, cerebellum, and heart, and congenital deafness have all been associated. Patients with much more frequent occurrence of fusion of only two adjacent cervical vertebrae may have osteoarthritis. (**Ref.** 5, p. 485)

265. **(A)** This is commonly associated with spina bifida. However, the usual explanation of cord fixation, adhesions, does not apply to the cases in which there is no defect in the lower spine and fails to account for the other anomalies commonly associated with the hindbrain malformation. (**Ref.** 5, pp. 480–482)

266. **(C)** Skull deformity similar to that of oxycephaly. All sutures are reportedly fused; the cranial configuration may be normal, but the brain is displaced upward. (**Ref.** 5, pp. 485–488)

267. **(C)** The facial appearance in general is similar. Proptosis, impaired ocular movement, and corneal drying have been attributed to elevated intracranial pressure but may be due at least partly to shallow orbits secondary to abnormal growth of facial bones. (**Ref.** 5, pp. 485–488)

268. (C) Maxillary hypoplasia, shortness of the upper lip, and prognathism. Both are autosomal dominant disorders. (**Ref.** 5, pp. 485–488)

269. (D) All the sutures are fused. Lambdoidal suture involvement produces flattening of the occiput and prominence of the parietal regions. (**Ref.** 5, pp. 485–488)

270. (A) Syndactyly is both osseous and cutaneous. The head is shortened in the anterior-posterior dimension, the forehead is prominent, and the occiput is flat. (**Ref.** 5, pp. 485–488)

8

Degenerative Diseases

DIRECTIONS (Questions 271–305): Each of the questions or incomplete statements below is followed by suggested answers or completions. Select the ONE that is BEST in each case.

271. In dystrophia myotonica
   A. weakness or myotonia generally occurs late
   B. facial and sternocleidomastoid muscles are usually severely affected
   C. fasciculation occurs in approximately one-half of all cases
   D. myotonia is generally relieved by cold
   E. myotonia is common in the thenar eminence and rare in the tongue

272. In McArdle's disease
   A. exercise relieves the weakness and stiffness but not the pain
   B. muscle phosphorylase is deficient
   C. muscle phosphorylase is excessive
   D. arm exercise with the arterial circulation occluded results in a normal rise of blood pyruvate but not of lactate
   E. arm exercise with the arterial circulation occluded results in a normal rise of blood lactate but not of pyruvate

273. Polymyositis
- **A.** shows weakness chronically, but not acutely
- **B.** includes hyperactive tendon reflexes early, hypoactive ones later
- **C.** features may include myocarditis and scleroderma
- **D.** shows a fall in blood gamma globulin; the sedimentation rate rises
- **E.** shows a decrease in serum transaminase

274. In Eaton-Lambert syndrome
- **A.** the amplitude of muscle action potentials evoked by nerve stimulation is markedly increased at first
- **B.** repetitive stimulation weakens the action potential
- **C.** there is an association with oat-cell carcinoma, other tumors, and other diseases; sometimes no other illness is found
- **D.** the deficit is not due to impaired release of acetylcholine
- **E.** cranial muscle weakness is prominent

275. In Huntington's chorea
- **A.** personality changes including depression and suicide may be prominent
- **B.** this hereditary disease typically has an insidious onset in adolescence
- **C.** certain aspects of the intellectual impairment are unique
- **D.** the neuropathology is not particularly characteristic
- **E.** the family history is invariably easy to obtain and greatly aids diagnosis

276. Tremor of extrapyramidal origin
- **A.** is slower and greater in amplitude than is tremor of thyrotoxicosis
- **B.** has been shown to have a very specific anatomic site of origin
- **C.** has been correlated with pathologic changes in the substantia nigra and globus pallidus; when these changes are present, tremor is invariably found, although its characteristics may vary
- **D.** is faster than that of anxiety
- **E.** is faster than that of intoxications

277. In cases of dyskinesia
   A. chorea suggests the lesser likelihood of a striatum lesion
   B. athetosis suggests a lesser likelihood of a striatal, pallidal, or cerebral cortex lesion
   C. patients with dystonia can inhibit and modify but not terminate the posturing
   D. ballismus usually is bilateral, although it sometimes affects only one limb
   E. tics are patterned, predictable, and reproducible

278. Muscle tone
   A. in chorea and athetosis is heightened in most muscle groups
   B. in rigidity appears to be due to impaired reciprocal inhibition of agonist and antagonist muscle groups
   C. in rigidity, EMG analysis shows continuing activity of only one of these two muscle groups throughout a movement
   D. rigidity has no effect on muscle power when tested carefully by dynamometry
   E. rigidity does not contribute to deformities

279. In extrapyramidal impairment of posture
   A. there is no loss of control of the center of gravity in the sagittal plane
   B. there is no loss of control of the center of gravity in the coronal plane
   C. pallidal degeneration is thought to be a factor
   D. righting reflexes are not involved
   E. vestibular reflexes are not involved

280. In patients with postencephalitic parkinsonism
   A. dystonic phenomena or tics are absent
   B. hemiplegia, bulbar, or ocular palsies may be found
   C. oculogyric crises may last for hours; the eyes deviate upward, not downward
   D. the parkinsonism is completely developed
   E. the parkinsonism progresses rapidly

281. In drug-induced parkinsonism
   A. adults are affected primarily and develop akinesia, rigidity, and a tremor
   B. children develop a similar picture, but dyskinetic movements are less pronounced
   C. centrally acting anticholinergic agents are usually ineffective
   D. akathisia is less frequently encountered
   E. symptoms occasionally persist for years after the drug is discontinued

282. In the treatment of parkinsonism
   A. anticholinergic therapy has been completely replaced by levodopa therapy
   B. certain phenothiazine derivatives have demonstrated antiparkinson activity
   C. amphetamine helps bradykinesia but not oculogyric crises
   D. all monoamine oxidase inhibitors must be avoided
   E. bromocriptine alone, usually 40–50 mg daily, is effective

283. In essential tremor
   A. there is a strong familial incidence with an autosomal dominant trait
   B. pathologic lesions have been found in the pallidum
   C. the dyskinesia is faster than that of parkinsonism, is worsened by volitional movement, and is often increased by alcohol
   D. propranolol is helpful in almost 90% of the cases
   E. sedatives have no effect

284. Senile tremor
   A. usually responds well to centrally acting anticholinergics
   B. is present first at rest and later with volitional movement
   C. has no known cause
   D. sedatives are of no value
   E. is associated with mild changes in muscle tone

285. In Sydenham's chorea
- **A.** cellular degeneration and varying degrees of arteritis are found
- **B.** lesions have been demonstrated in the basal ganglia and cortex, but not in the brain stem
- **C.** the basal ganglia and cerebellar systems have been the only significant loci of disease
- **D.** onset of symptoms is usually abrupt
- **E.** muscle tone is normal

286. In Huntington's chorea
- **A.** there is a single dominant autosomal gene expressed primarily in males
- **B.** phenothiazines or reserpine may be helpful
- **C.** dancing gait is a prominent feature, although the uppers are more often involved than the lowers
- **D.** tetrabenazine is of no value
- **E.** haloperidol does not help

287. In the clinical picture of athetosis
- **A.** muscles innervated by cranial nerves are infrequently involved
- **B.** abnormal limb postures are present; intellectual impairment is often found
- **C.** hypotonia is almost constantly present; weakness is not usually found
- **D.** reflexes are invariably normal
- **E.** limbs are involved, especially proximally

288. In dystonia musculorum deformans
- **A.** mentation, muscle tone, strength, and reflexes are all normal
- **B.** the age of onset parallels that of athetosis
- **C.** anticholinergic drugs, levodopa, and excision of a minute thalamic nuclear lesion via a single surgical procedure are usually all effective
- **D.** speech is unimpaired
- **E.** plasma dopamine beta-hydroxylase activity is depressed

289. In spasmodic torticollis
   A. facial and brachial muscles are not involved
   B. although its pathophysiology and pathology are unknown, its clinical course is consistently progressive
   C. congenital ocular muscle imbalance and defective cervical spine or musculature have been considered as causes
   D. sensory biofeedback is of no value
   E. the onset typically occurs in adolescence

290. Hemiballism does not occur
   A. in tumors
   B. soon after a cerebrovascular episode has taken place
   C. after attempted thalamotomy for other extrapyramidal disorders
   D. in infectious disease
   E. in subdural hematoma and subarachnoid hemorrhage

291. In idiopathic orthostatic hypotension
   A. impotence, constipation, and urinary urgency or retention are infrequent
   B. steroids are not used
   C. death may occur 5 to 15 years from onset
   D. support stockings are not used
   E. L-dopa is of consistent value

292. In Shy-Drager syndrome
   A. peripheral neuropathy is frequently found
   B. autonomic insufficiency of Wernicke's encephalopathy, tabes, syringomyelia, and diabetic neuropathy must be considered
   C. orthostatic hypotension of myocardial infarction, aortic stenosis, or GI hemorrhage can be excluded by the development of tachycardia and the absence of sweating
   D. familial hyperbradykininism features other signs of autonomic dysfunction
   E. posterior fossa mass lesions produce other signs of autonomic dysfunction

293. In adynamia episodica hereditaria
   A. the serum potassium is low during the attack
   B. calcium gluconate may aggravate the attack
   C. the age of onset is usually less than 10 years

    D. insulin may provoke an attack
    E. acetazolamide increases the severity of the episode

294. Temporal arteritis
    A. is not associated with inflammation of the internal carotid artery
    B. is self-limited but should be treated as early as possible
    C. produces giant cell arteritis of extracranial arteries, which may coexist with giant cell arteritis of the CNS; the latter does not occur alone
    D. is often associated with polymyalgia rheumatica, in which weakness is usually prominent
    E. has a clinical course of steady progression unless interrupted by steroid administration

295. Collagen disease
    A. involves the CNS but not muscles
    B. involves the peripheral nervous system
    C. involves muscles but not the CNS
    D. is becoming less frequent
    E. does not involve the spinal cord

296. Polyarteritis nodosa
    A. produces inflammation of small- and medium-sized arteries, excluding their adventitia; occasionally veins are involved
    B. is associated with asthma, serum sickness, and reactions to sulfa drugs
    C. usually begins in the second decade of life
    D. may be associated with positive tests for syphilis and trichinosis; leukopenia with an inconstant eosinophilia is found
    E. neuropathy is the least common of all neurologic complications

297. In periarteritis nodosa
    A. thrombosis and hemorrhage occur
    B. multiple neuropathies are uncommon
    C. the autonomic nervous system is not involved
    D. keratitis and deafness occur, provided that the CSF Wassermann reaction is positive
    E. the course is differentiated from that of multiple sclerosis by the absence of remissions

298. Temporal arteritis
   A. is pathologically similar to polyarteritis nodosa
   B. usually begins in the third decade of life
   C. produces blindness due to hemorrhage of the central retinal artery
   D. can be diagnosed by biopsy of nerve or muscle, but not of testicle
   E. causes death, usually by renal or CNS involvement

299. Preferred treatment of paralysis agitans is
   A. medical treatment with L-dopa and carbidopa
   B. surgical treatment of the older patient with bilateral disease
   C. trihexyphenidyl, usually 20–25 mg daily in divided doses
   D. atropine and prochlorperazine
   E. diphenhydramine, 50 mg daily

300. Tetany
   A. includes the triad of carpopedal spasm, laryngospasm, and convulsions
   B. causes convulsions less often than the other symptoms
   C. produces muscle spasm, which may last for as long as an hour
   D. usually produces a normal EMG
   E. causes prolonged expiratory stridor

301. In Dejerine-Sottas disease
   A. thickened peripheral nerves are found
   B. onset is usually in middle age
   C. nerve conduction velocities are not appreciably impaired
   D. the CSF protein is normal
   E. there are no sensory abnormalities

302. In familial dysautonomia, degenerative changes do not occur in
   A. reticular formation of the brain stem
   B. spinal cord
   C. celiac plexus
   D. muscles
   E. dorsal root ganglia

303. The Riley-Day syndrome
  A. does not usually shorten life
  B. includes episodes of hypertension and hyperpyrexia
  C. does not usually include seizures
  D. does not cause postural hypotension
  E. shows no changes in tongue papillae

304. Muscular dystrophy (facioscapulohumeral type)
  A. most often occurs in early childhood
  B. may be present for 50 years without preventing the ability to walk
  C. often involves ocular and tongue muscles
  D. often includes pseudohypertrophy
  E. often produces contractures

305. In syringobulbia
  A. atrophy and fasciculations of the tongue do not occur
  B. facial loss of pain and temperature usually do not occur
  C. development may be rapid
  D. dysphagia does not occur
  E. pharyngeal weakness does not occur

DIRECTIONS (Questions 306–320): The set of lettered headings below is followed by a list of numbered words or phrases. For each numbered word or phrase select
  A. if the item is associated with A only
  B. if the item is associated with B only
  C. if the item is associated with both A and B
  D. if the item is associated with neither A nor B

Questions 306–320:

  A. Parkinsonism
  B. Pseudoparkinsonism
  C. Both
  D. Neither

306. Arteriosclerotic parkinsonism

307. État lacunaire

308. Extensive involvement of the substantia nigra

309. Greater involvement of the globus pallidus, along with lesions of the brain stem and cerebral cortex

310. In one report, tremor was the presenting complaint in 70% of cases

311. "Gegenhalten"

312. Abnormal plantar responses are usually found

313. Gait disturbance is the most frequent initial complaint

314. Early complaints often include dysarthria, dysphagia, and emotional incontinence

315. Stepwise, more rapid course

316. Good tolerance of anticholinergic treatment

317. Good tolerance of dopaminergic treatment

318. Impairment of downward gaze early

319. Total ophthalmoplegia

320. Head tilt backward

DIRECTIONS (Questions 321–330): Each group of questions below consists of lettered headings followed by a list of numbered words or statements. For each numbered word or statement, select the ONE lettered heading that is most closely associated with it. Each lettered heading may be selected once, more than once, or not at all.

Questions 321–325:

A. Relentlessly progressive, gradual course; generally no sensory loss, incontinence, nor ocular weakness; upper and lower motor neuron signs
B. Slow course; no upper motor neuron signs
C. Sensory symptoms; no lower motor neuron signs in legs; MRI or myelogram positive
D. No weakness nor atrophy
E. Onset in youth; strictly focal; no upper motor neuron signs

321. Compression myelopathy due to cervical spondylosis or extramedullary tumor

322. Amyotrophic lateral sclerosis

323. Post-polio progressive muscular atrophy

324. Benign focal amyotrophy

325. Benign fasciculations

Questions 326–330:

A. Most common focal torsion dystonia; usually starts in adulthood and remains limited to this region; occasionally spreads to involve vocal cords and one or both arms

B. Occurs in many diseases; combination of clonazepam and valproate often effective in some syndromes

C. Vocal tics, obscene words or gestures

D. Most often found in patients with perinatal brain injury; involves limbs (distal and proximal), trunk, neck, face, and tongue; no satisfactory treatment

E. Increased blinking followed by focal contractions of orbicularis oculi and often involvement of other muscles innervated by facial nerve; further spread involves jaw muscles and is also called "blepharospasm-plus"; may cause functional blindness

326. Athetosis

327. Myoclonus

328. Spasmodic torticollis

329. Meige's syndrome

330. Gilles de la Tourette's syndrome

Answers and Discussion

271. (B) The face is expressionless, the eyelids often droop and the cheeks are sunken. Most patients are identified by the combination of myotonia, dystrophic weakness, and cataracts. Cold weather produces stiffness. The tongue is involved. Fasciculations do not occur. (**Ref.** 5, pp. 714–718)

272. (B) In this recessive disorder, glycogen accumulates because of the enzyme deficiency. There is failure of lactate production on ischemic exercise. Exercise produces cramps. (**Ref.** 4, p. 438)

273. (C) Acute cases exhibit fever and a polymorphonuclear leukocytosis in the blood. The onset often follows a viral infection which may initially sensitize lymphocytes and cause muscle damage, followed by further sensitization. Tendon reflexes disappear. Weakness is present in both acute and chronic forms. (**Ref.** 4, pp. 428–430)

274. (C) The syndrome may be defined in terms of the EMG. Microelectric studies indicate that the defect is due to impaired release of acetylcholine at the nerve terminals. Initial nerve stimulation reduces the amplitude of muscle action potential; repetitive stimulation increases it. (**Ref.** 9, p. 2058)

275. (A) Clinical diagnosis depends not on any distinguishing feature of the dementia but rather on the choreiform movements that accompany or precede it. There are multiple causes of chorea; progressive dementia and emotional disturbances strongly suggest

Huntington's disease. The disease is readily apparent if a positive family history is obtained. Peak age at onset is 40 years. Primarily, the striatum and cerebral cortex show loss of neurons and reactive gliosis. (**Ref.** 9, pp. 2147–2148)

276. (A)   Although the varieties or tremor can be correlated with various disorders, its exact anatomic site is unknown; there may be multiple pathologic sites. (**Ref.** 9, pp. 2141–2142)

277. (E)   In athetosis and chorea, many areas have shown pathologic changes, some more often than others. The situation in dystonia is less fully defined; in ballismus, it is the most specific. (**Ref.** 9, pp. 2141–2150)

278. (B)   Chorea and athetosis may show normal tone or hypotonia; in extrapyramidal disorders, a variety of muscle tension states is found. In rigidity, EMG recordings reveal that the agonist and antagonist muscles contract simultaneously, even when the patient attempts to relax. (**Ref.** 9, p. 2143)

279. (C)   These abnormalities are felt to be due to defects in righting reflexes, vestibular reflexes, and proprioceptor mechanisms. Postural reflexes can be tested by pulling the standing patient backward or forward toward the examiner with a quick tug on the shoulders; one should be ready to catch the patient. (**Ref.** 9, p. 2143)

280. (B)   In most cases of secondary parkinsonism, neurologic abnormalities involving other areas of the nervous system are found. Affected patients may also have dystonia, chorea, tics, or behavioral disorders. Most often, these parkinsonian syndromes remain stable or improved. (**Ref.** 9, p. 2144)

281. (A)   Several extrapyramidal syndromes have occurred; in most cases, anticholinergic treatment can prevent or minimize the symptoms. Unfortunately, one of the syndromes, tardive dyskinesia, may be irreversible. (**Ref.** 9, p. 2144)

282. (B)   Parsidol is one such drug. A common method of management utilizes the centrally acting anticholinergics either alone or

in combination with L-dopa; each is given gradually to tolerance. Some advocate beginning with the anticholinergics and amantadine; L-dopa is added later. Selegiline has been added in recent years. (**Ref.** 9, pp. 2145–2146)

283. (A) Differentiation from parkinsonism is particularly important because of the difference in prognosis and management. Beta-adrenergic blocking agents are useful in some patients with essential tremor. A small amount of ethanol temporarily reduces the tremor. Primidone sometimes is helpful. (**Ref.** 9, p. 2147)

284. (C) It is assumed that degenerative factors affect connections between the cerebellar and extrapyramidal systems. It is now felt that essential tremor, familiar tremor, and senile tremor are the same; the last has a late-life onset. No specific pathologic condition in the nervous system has been reported in this condition. (**Ref.** 9, p. 2147)

285. (A) No specific pathologic or anatomic changes have been found. Scattered vasculitic lesions have been found in the cortex, basal ganglia, cerebellum, and brain stem. Clinically, recurrence is found in almost one-third of the patients. (**Ref.** 9, p. 2149)

286. (B) There is no specific therapy; the disease is progressive; unaffected individuals rarely transmit it. In management, it is important to counsel the family with regard to genetic implications and also because of the enormous family stress created by the patient's mental symptoms. Pre-synaptic dopamine-depleting agents (reserpine and tetrabenazine) may help. (**Ref.** 9, p. 2148)

287. (B) The athetotic movements are superimposed on these abnormal postures; however, details of the clinical picture vary. It has been suggested that athetosis is the expression of torsion dystonia caused by basal ganglia damage at an early age. Involvement includes face and tongue. Speech is impaired. (**Ref.** 9, p. 2152)

288. (A) The condition is rare, its cause is unknown, and the course is extremely variable; therefore, evaluation of the efficacy of treatment is difficult. Thus, patients with this condition should not undergo surgical treatment for it unless they are well aware of the risks, have had an adequate trial of pharmacologic agents, and have intractable, disabling symptoms. No drug has been consistently effective and surgical procedures are generally multiple, when they are attempted. (**Ref.** 9, pp. 2149–2150)

289. (C) Investigation in a given case includes a search for ocular and vertebral abnormalities, psychiatric illness, and other neurologic conditions; usually, no cause of these movements is found. Pharmacologic therapy, sensory feedback therapy, and dorsal column stimulation may help. Surgical section of the spinal accessory nerve produces inconsistent relief. The condition usually begins in adulthood. (**Ref.** 9, p. 2150)

290. (E) The condition is due to involvement of the contralateral subthalamic nucleus, usually by a vascular lesion. Severe movements can be exhausting but can be controlled with drugs such as reserpine or antipsychotic agents. (**Ref.** 9, p. 2148)

291. (C) Oral sympathomimetics are occasionally administered. Support stockings and steroids are used. (**Ref.** 9, pp. 2106–2107)

292. (B) Other neurologic illnesses to be considered frequently include sensory deficits in the limbs and other manifestations of peripheral neuropathy. In Shy-Drager syndrome, other changes are reduced sweating, iris atrophy, impaired eye movements, sexual impotence, and bladder and bowel dysfunction. (**Ref.** 9, pp. 2106–2107)

293. (C) Diuretics tend to reduce the number of attacks; administration of potassium chloride increases them. Attacks may be terminated by administration of calcium gluconate, glucose, and insulin. (**Ref.** 5, p. 723)

294. (B) This is usually limited to the temporal arteries but occasionally involves other arteries of the head and, rarely, even involves arteries elsewhere in the body. Prednisone therapy helps to shorten the course and prevents blindness in the unaffected eye if started while symptoms are unilateral. In polymyalgia there is no weakness. (**Ref.** 5, pp. 888–889)

295. (B) At least some of these lesions occur in all of the major collagen diseases. Some of these diseases seem due to the deposition of circulating immune complexes within the vessel walls and some may be due to persistent viral infection. Brain, cord, peripheral nerves, and muscles are involved. (**Ref.** 5, p. 885)

296. (B) Because of (B), plus deposition of antigen-antibody complexes in arterial walls, etc., anaphylactic hypersensitivity has been suggested as an etiologic factor. This hypothesis was supported by work done years ago in which repeated injection of horse serum reproduced the lesions in rabbits. There is widespread panarteritis. Most cases are in the third and fourth decades of life. (**Ref.** 5, pp. 885–888)

297. (A) The diffuse panarteritis affects the peripheral, central, and autonomic nervous systems. The adventitia, vasa vasorum, media, elastic membrane, and intima are all involved. Remissions may occur. (**Ref.** 5, pp. 885–888)

298. (A) In this disorder the inflammatory reaction is more severe and there are multinucleated giant cells in the media. The syndrome of polymyalgia rheumatica may overlap with that of temporal arteritis. Temporal arteritis usually begins in the sixth to eighth decades of life. Blindness is presumably due to thrombosis of the central retinal artery. (**Ref.** 5, pp. 888–889)

299. (A) Administration of L-dopa and carbidopa, alone or in combination with other antiparkinson medications, is the preferred method. These drugs are optimal during the first three years of use; later, their effectiveness somewhat declines. Surgical therapy has been used less since the advent of L-dopa therapy. Experimental transplant procedures are still being attempted. (**Ref.** 5, pp. 668–670)

300. (A) The differential diagnosis concerns the various causes of hypocalcemia and alkalosis. It also occurs in hypomagnesemia and occasionally represents a primary neural abnormality. EMG is abnormal. (**Ref.** 5, p. 732)

301. (A) A systemic biochemical abnormality has been found. The condition is recessively inherited and is present in childhood with progressive limb weakness, stocking-and-glove impairment of sensation, and generalized hyporeflexia. Nerve conduction velocities are usually less than 10 m per second; CSF protein is elevated. (**Ref.** 5, pp. 605–606)

302. (D) However, in some cases, examination of the central and peripheral nervous systems has been entirely normal. Decreased neuronal counts have been found in cervical sympathetic ganglia, sympathetic preganglionic spinal cord neurons, and parasympathetic sphenopalatine ganglia. (**Ref.** 5, pp. 770–772)

303. (B) Diagnosis is made by the clinical picture occurring in early life and the increase in urinary homovanilic acid. Hyperresponsiveness to sympathetic drugs suggests a denervation-type supersensitivity. Forty % of patients have seizures in early life; fewer than 10% have subsequent seizure disorders. Postural hypotension occurs. Fungiform papillae of the tongue are absent. (**Ref.** 5, pp. 770–772)

304. (B) Classification into Duchenne type, facioscapulohumeral type, and limb-girdle type at least present a certain degree of validity in prognosis. Although the symptoms and signs suggest a single disease entity, families with similar clinical manifestations may be separated by differing pathologic and EMG features. This disorder usually begins in adolescence; ocular and tongue muscles are spared. (**Ref.** 5, pp. 713–714)

305. (C) This may occur alone but usually is found in combination with cervical syringomyelia. Rarely, the syrinx may extend even higher in the brainstem or into the centrum semiovale as a syringocephalus. Dysphagia, pharyngeal, and palatal weakness occur. (**Ref.** 5, pp. 687–690)

306. (B) The underlying substrate of cerebrovascular disease. However, only rarely is there a history of a major stroke preceding this onset. (**Ref.** 5, pp. 658–664)

307. (B) Multiple small cerebral infarctions are diffusely present. Onset of symptoms is usually insidious, with most cases beginning in the seventh decade of life. (**Ref.** 5, pp. 658–664)

308. (A) Substantia nigra involvement in pseudoparkinsonism is much less marked. There is neuronal loss and depigmentation, especially in the zona compacta. (**Ref.** 5, pp. 658–664)

309. (B) This is part of the characteristically diffuse neuronal cell loss. Multiple small vessel occlusions are not infrequently found throughout the brain. (**Ref.** 5, pp. 658–664)

310. (A) Tremor is rare in pseudoparkinsonism. However, on questioning, many patients recall other symptoms as having been present for years preceding the tremor. (**Ref.** 5, pp. 658–664)

311. (B) The limb stiffens in response to contact, and a sense of resistance is noted with attempted change of position. (**Ref.** 5, p. 664)

312. (B) Reflexes are generally hyperactive; the snout reflex is usually found. Palmo-mental reflexes are also found. Masked fascies are relatively rare. (**Ref.** 5, p. 664; **Ref.** 9, p. 2145)

313. (D) Progressive intellectual deficits occasionally are early signs. The gait problem includes short steps, "freezing," and unsteadiness on turning. (**Ref.** 9, p. 2145)

314. (B) Pseudobulbar phenomena sometimes are early manifestations. Vascular parkinsonism may appear in middle life or old age. (**Ref.** 9, p. 2145; **Ref.** 5, p. 664)

315. (B) Treatment is of limited effectiveness. Tolerance of the usual antiparkinson drugs, whether anticholinergic or dopaminergic, is poor. (**Ref.** 5, p. 664)

316. (A) There must be careful dosage titration against side effects. Several drugs are available; there is little reason, aside from personal preference, for choosing one rather than another. (**Ref.** 5, p. 665)

317. (A) Adjunctive medications include amantadine, antidepressants, and diphenhydramine. Bromocriptine may also be useful but has additional side effects. Selegiline (Deprenyl) has been used more recently. (**Ref.** 19, pp. 859–861; **Ref.** 5, p. 668)

318. (D) This is an early sign of progressive supranuclear palsy. In addition, the patient cannot flex the neck to use the head. (**Ref.** 5, pp. 671–673)

319. (D) In progressive supranuclear palsy, this follows vertical gaze palsy. Characteristically, ocular movement is preserved in oculocephalic maneuvers, indicating that the ocular palsy is supranuclear in origin. (**Ref.** 5, pp. 671–673)

320. (D) In progressive supranuclear palsy, intense rigidity, especially of the posterior cervical muscles, may result in fixed hyperextension of the head. The cause of the condition is unknown. (**Ref.** 5, pp. 671–673)

321. (C) Treatable but results vary. (**Ref.** 9, p. 2156)

322. (A) No medication known to be beneficial. (**Ref.** 9, p. 2156)

323. (B) Progressive weakness years after a severe attack of polio; overall, prognosis generally good. (**Ref.** 9, pp. 2199–2200)

324. (E) Slowly progressive; no involvement of sensory pathways. (**Ref.** 9, p. 2156; **Ref.** 5, p. 680)

325. (D) EMG is normal. (**Ref.** 9, p. 2156; **Ref.** 5, pp. 409–411)

326. (D) Usually from hypoxic damage. (**Ref.** 9, p. 2152)

327. (B) One form of progressive encephalopathy with myoclonus is responsive to biotin. (**Ref.** 9, p. 2151)

328. (A) Many patients improve moderately with drug therapy. (**Ref.** 9, p. 2150)

329. (E) Bright light aggravates the blepharospasm. Botulinum toxin injections help. (**Ref.** 9, p. 2150)

330. (C) Haloperidol, clonazepam, and clonidine help. (**Ref.** 9, pp. 2151–2152)

9

Myelinopathies

DIRECTIONS (Questions 331–332): Each of the questions or incomplete statements below is followed by suggested answers or completions. Select the ONE that is BEST in each case.

331. The spinal fluid findings in multiple sclerosis
  - **A.** are generally pathognomonic
  - **B.** are not generally pathognomonic
  - **C.** not infrequently include a marked pleocytosis
  - **D.** usually include a decrease in sugar
  - **E.** usually include an increase in total protein

332. In multiple sclerosis
  - **A.** convulsions occur in approximately 20% of cases
  - **B.** visual loss is generally unilateral
  - **C.** headache and aphasia are not unusual
  - **D.** neurogenic atrophy is not uncommon
  - **E.** internuclear ophthalmoplegia, hearing loss, and tinnitus are common

---

DIRECTIONS (Questions 333–339): The group of questions below consists of a list of lettered headings followed by a list of numbered words, phrases, or statements. For each numbered word, phrase, or statement, select the ONE lettered heading that is most closely associated with it. Each lettered heading may be selected once, more than once, or not at all.

Questions 333–339:

    A. Krabbe's disease
    B. Metachromatic leukoencephalopathy
    C. Schilder's disease
    D. Pelizaeus-Merzbacher disease

333. The pathogenesis felt to be same as that of multiple sclerosis

334. Islands of preserved myelin

335. Perivascular "globoid" cells

336. Granular material, possibly a defect in sulfatide metabolism in the brain, nerves, kidney, and liver

337. Exact diagnosis is possible in life without craniotomy

338. Abnormal lipoid products are also found in the pituitary and testes

339. Arylsulfatase A activity is said to be deficient

DIRECTIONS (Questions 340–343): The set of lettered headings below is followed by a list of numbered words or phrases. For each numbered word or phrase select

    A. if the item is associated with A only
    B. if the item is associated with B only
    C. if the item is associated with both A and B
    D. if the item is associated with neither A nor B

Questions 340–343:

    A. Adrenoleukodystrophy
    B. Sudanophilic leukodystrophy
    C. Both
    D. Neither

340. Dysmyelinating primarily or only

341. Myelinoclastic primarily or only

342. Three subtypes proposed

343. Manifestations of Addison's disease tend to precede those of Schilder's disease

Answers and Discussion

331. (B) There is currently no single completely pathognomonic laboratory test for this disease. The finding of typical changes in CSF IgG, when coupled with the history and the clinical examination, appears to be the most valuable diagnostic aid. The presence of oligoclonal or polyclonal bands is another aid in diagnosis. (**Ref.** 5, pp. 753–755)

332. (B) In Devic's disease (a possible variant of multiple sclerosis) the visual loss is bilateral. Devic's disease has been considered a syndrome because it may occur in acute disseminated encephalomyelitis, systemic lupus erythematosus, or sarcoidosis. Convulsions, decreased hearing, and tinnitus all occur in multiple sclerosis but are uncommon. (**Ref.** 9, p. 2215; **Ref.** 5, pp. 750–751)

333. (C) This is considered myelinoclastic. What became known as "Schilder's disease" was a heterogeneous group of disorders that included demylinating diseases related to multiple sclerosis, inflammatory disorders with secondary demyelination, and progressive genetic metabolic disorders affecting myelin metabolism. (**Ref.** 5, pp. 513–516)

334. (D) This condition starts in infancy; the course is prolonged. This disease was also set apart by X-linked inheritance. (**Ref.** 5, pp. 513–516)

335. **(A)** Psychomotor arrest and regression occur in mid-infancy; there is increased CSF protein; the course is progressive. Fevers, seizures, vomiting, and optic atrophy also occur. (**Ref.** 5, pp. 513–516)

336. **(B)** Sulfatide, because of enzyme deficiency, is not broken down into cerebroside. Sulfatase A appears to be the major defective enzyme involved. Therefore, sulfated lipid levels increase. (**Ref.** 5, pp. 513–516, 527–530)

337. **(B)** For example, the nitrocatechol sulfate test is useful. Clinically, metachromatic leukodystrophy resembles many other diseases. (**Ref.** 5, pp. 513–516, 527–530)

338. **(B)** Sulfatide is also found in renal tubes. There is a profound leukodystrophy in the CNS that tends to spare the arcuate fibers. (**Ref.** 5, pp. 513–516, 527–530)

339. **(B)** However, administration of enzyme produces no single change in the disease picture or course. No specific therapy is available. (**Ref.** 5, pp. 513–516, 527–530)

340. **(C)** Widespread dysmyelination occurs in sudanophilic leukodystrophy; some myelinoclastic areas are found in adrenoleukodystrophy, but the main process appears to be demyelination. Dysmyelination suggests problems in the formation or maintenance of myelin. Demyelination (myelinoclastic) suggests normal myelin formation, with subsequent damage to it. (**Ref.** 5, p. 513)

341. **(D)** Peripheral nerve demyelination is found in adrenoleukodystrophy. Adrenoleukodystrophy also has X-linked inheritance. (**Ref.** 5, p. 513)

342. **(B)** Validity of the three subtypes is doubtful. This heterogeneous group of unclassified leukodystrophies is sometimes also called "orthochromatic" or "unclassified leukodystrophies." (**Ref.** 5, p. 513)

343. (A) Unfortunately, correction of the Addison state does not alter the process of the diffuse sclerosis. Another X-linked leukodystrophy with adrenal involvement is termed "adrenomyeloneuropathy." (**Ref.** 5, p. 515)

10

Convulsive and Other Paroxysmal Disorders

DIRECTIONS (Questions 344–357): Each of the questions or incomplete statements below is followed by suggested answers or completions. Select the ONE that is BEST in each case.

344. In epilepsy, valproic acid
   A. is not readily absorbed from the GI tract
   B. may have an effect on the metabolism of gamma-aminobutyric acid
   C. when administered concomitantly with phenobarbital, may depress the phenobarbital plasma concentration
   D. when administered concomitantly with phenytoin sodium, consistently raises the phenytoin plasma concentration
   E. frequently produces hepatic failure, especially in adults

345. Syncope may occur
  A. after coughing or voiding
  B. on compression of the carotid sinus
  C. on sudden exposure to cold
  D. B and C but not A
  E. A and B but not C

346. In tic douloureux
  A. the pain is almost constant
  B. the eye may close and have tears
  C. one can usually demonstrate small areas of hypalgesia
  D. disseminated sclerosis is present in about 25% of the cases
  E. Dilantin is of no value

347. All of the following are postulated mechanisms of headache except
  A. dysfunction of extracranial arteries
  B. traction on intracranial vessels
  C. pressure on cranial nerves
  D. pressure on cerebral parenchyma
  E. cervical spondylosis

348. Cough syncope
  A. occurs equally often in men and women, regardless of cause
  B. is not more likely to occur in brain tumors or in cerebral stenotic arterial disease
  C. often occurs with chronic lung disease in the adult; with pertussis in children
  D. does not occur in recumbency
  E. may be preceded by focal neurologic symptoms

349. In micturition syncope
  A. women and men are affected equally often
  B. there may be a situation converse to that of the paraplegic's paroxysmal hypertension during bladder distention
  C. the episode resembles that following paracentesis removal of a small amount of ascitic fluid
  D. postsyncopal confusion occurs
  E. postsyncopal weakness occurs

350. Ménière's disease
  A. is one of the most frequent causes of nonvertiginous dizziness
  B. usually begins in middle life and includes tinnitus
  C. causes hearing loss that is usually bilateral
  D. causes bouts of vertigo lasting for up to one hour
  E. rarely "burns out"

351. On testing of the hearing loss in Ménière's disease
  A. low-frequency, pure tone impairment is found
  B. tone decay is found
  C. the SISI score is very low
  D. recruitment is absent
  E. speech discrimination is good

352. In vestibular neuronitis
  A. nystagmus is usually absent
  B. most patients remain very ill for 72 to 96 hours
  C. the patient often awakens one morning after a viral infection with vertigo, nausea, and ataxia, veering toward the involved side
  D. hearing is impaired
  E. recurrence takes place at variable intervals in younger patients

353. In benign positional vertigo
  A. attacks depend upon the assumption of certain positions; between episodes, slight dizziness is usually present
  B. any pathophysiologic theory must explain the latent period before symptom production
  C. the vertigo is severe and lasts for 10 to 15 minutes
  D. caloric tests are frequently abnormal
  E. in most cases, symptoms last for two to three years

354. In chronic orthostatic hypotension
  A. typically, reflex arteriolar constriction is adequate but venous return is not
  B. the pulse rate increases rapidly in an attempt to compensate
  C. diabetic neuropathy or tabes dorsalis should be sought
  D. pallor and sweating occur
  E. nausea occurs

355. In vasovagal attack
   A. pallor and sweating do not occur
   B. peripheral vasodilatation, especially in the muscles, is the final event
   C. absence of immediate muscular activity and a failure to increase cardiac output help lead to a reduction in cerebral blood flow
   D. pupillary dilatation and bradycardia occur early
   E. headaches and confusion are part of the presyncopal phase

356. In Adams-Stokes syndrome
   A. attacks are usually related to posture
   B. convulsive movements occur
   C. syncope occurs during asystole, but ventricular fibrillation does not
   D. prodromal signs are present
   E. pupillary dilatation does not occur

357. In testing the carotid sinuses as a possible cause of syncope
   A. compression of the carotid vessels per se can complicate evaluation of results
   B. atropine usually has no effect on the carotid sinus response
   C. the most common response is a vasodepressor, one without bradycardia
   D. posture plays no role
   E. permanent demand pacemakers may be considered as therapy in the case of a positive test per se

---

DIRECTIONS (Questions 358–376): Each group of questions below consists of a list of lettered headings followed by a list of numbered words, phrases, or statements. For each numbered word, phrase, or statement, select the ONE lettered heading that is most closely associated with it. Each lettered heading may be selected once, more than once, or not at all.

Questions 358–363:

   A. Cataplexy
   B. Sleep paralysis

    C. Hypnagogic hallucinations
    D. Parasomnia
    E. Narcolepsy
    F. Somnambulism

358. Unable to move on awakening

359. Sudden loss of posture with preservation of consciousness

360. Specifically alters vision or hearing

361. Performing complex activities while being unaware of them

362. When symptomatic, is usually due to a lesion in the region of the third ventricle

363. A variety of stupor

Questions 364–369:

    A. Drop attacks
    B. "Television" epilepsy
    C. Jacksonian epilepsy
    D. Epilepsia partialis continua
    E. Temporal lobe epilepsy
    F. Todd's paralysis

364. Can be confirmed during EEG with flicker activation

365. Characteristically begins unilaterally

366. Ascribed to brain stem ischemia

367. Déjà vu, uncinate, and gustatory phenomena

368. Weakness for several hours up to one to two days

369. Remains confined to a limited part of the body

Questions 370–376:

    A. Infantile spasms
    B. Gelastic epilepsy
    C. Petit mal
    D. Grand mal
    E. Psychomotor seizures

370. Laughter as one of the manifestations of the attack

371. Characteristically associated with hypsarrhythmia

372. Associated with phenylketonuria or hypoglycemia; lightning-fast movements

373. Control of seizures by steroids

374. Regularly precipitated by hyperventilation

375. Focus typically in one temporal lobe

376. Precipitated by subconvulsive doses of convulsants, over-hydration, and pitressin

Answers and Discussion

344. (B) This effect may be produced, for example, by competitive inhibition of GABA-transaminase. Valproic acid is effective against a variety of seizure types. (**Ref.** 9, pp. 2226–2227; **Ref.** 5, pp. 801–802)

345. (E) Other causes include disturbances of heart rate and rhythm, emotional stress, and postural hypotension. Postural hypotension occasionally results from rare degenerative diseases affecting the autonomic nervous system (idiopathic orthostatic hypotension), sometimes in association with multisystemic atrophy (Shy-Drager syndrome). (**Ref.** 4, pp. 195–196)

346. (B) The attacks are typically brief, severe, and often precipitated by stimulation of a "trigger spot." Carbamazepine has been effective; dilantin less so. Surgical section, by causing analgesia of the cornea, may lead to neuropathic keratitis. Microvascular decompression procedures (posterior fossa) are also used. (**Ref.** 4, p. 63; **Ref.** 5, pp. 419–420)

347. (D) Headache may also be referred from cranial structures (eye, nasal sinuses, etc.) or even from thoracic or abdominal viscera. Psychogenic headaches can have a large variety of manifestations; they may be a symptom of underlying anxiety or depression; reassurance, tranquilizers, or antidepressants often help. (**Ref.** 4, p. 215)

348. (C) This condition usually follows vigorous coughing. Its cause has been attributed to a reduction in cardiac output or to a sudden elevation in CSF pressure. A similar mechanism is thought to occur in "weightlifting syncope." Emotional fainting seems more common in women; fainting after pain, more common in men. **(Ref. 5, pp. 18–19)**

349. (B) Suggested pathogenetic mechanisms have included peripheral vasodilation and the Valsalva effect. The anoxic syncope is sometimes followed by brief tonic or clonic movements and rarely by generalized convulsions. **(Ref. 5, pp. 792–793)**

350. (B) This condition is said to be the most common cause of true vertigo; patients with pseudo-Ménière's syndrome also eventually tend to develop the complete symptom triad. Recurrent endolymphatic hypertension (hydrops) is believed to cause the episode. **(Ref. 9, p. 2119)**

351. (A) The deafness on testing appears to be more typical of sense organ (cochlear) damage than of nerve trunk (retrocochlear) damage. In addition, the abnormal vestibular findings often parallel the hearing loss. Loudness recruitment is almost always present. **(Ref. 5, pp. 806–807)**

352. (C) This was previously called "acute labyrinthitis"; current etiologic theories favor a viral neuronitis or a postinfectious demyelinating reaction. This may occur as a single bout or may recur repeatedly over months or years. **(Ref. 9, p. 2123; Ref. 5, p. 426)**

353. (B) The several reported causes of this and of "malignant" positional vertigo include labyrinthine disorder, trauma, infection, vascular occlusion, prolonged systemic illness, toxins, and even brain tumor. Repetitively producing the vertigo each day may give prolonged relief. Each episode typically lasts less than one minute and the episodes usually remit in less than one month from the onset but they may recur. **(Ref. 9, p. 2123)**

354. (C) A variety of autonomic malfunctions may occur; the condition has also been associated with a rare form of Parkinson-like syndrome. In treating orthostatic hypotension, the use of monoamine oxidase inhibitors may be potentially hazardous in those patients who are subject to denervation supersensitivity. (**Ref.** 9, pp. 2106–2107)

355. **(C)** In this condition, also called "vasodepressor syncope," there are autonomic manifestations in the presyncopal stage and other symptoms in the postsyncopal stage. This is the most common cause of fainting. (**Ref.** 9, p. 2074)

356. **(B)** In this condition, fainting typically occurs in association with bradycardia, but other arrhythmias also occur; asystole may cause syncope and, if prolonged, convulsive movements and confusion. The most common cardiac causes of syncope are probably the cardiac arrhythmias, including Stokes-Adams attacks. (**Ref.** 5, pp. 16–20)

357. **(A)** Many patients, especially older ones, show bradycardia and hypotension during carotid sinus massage; the condition is probably related to atherosclerosis of the carotid sinus region. Bradycardia or cardiac arrest are more common than drop in blood pressure. (**Ref.** 5, p. 18; **Ref.** 4, p. 196)

358. **(B)** This type is also called "postdormitial"; sleep paralysis occuring at the onset of sleep is called "predormitial." The patient is fully conscious during the episode. He usually believes that the paralysis has lasted for many minutes, but the actual duration is much briefer. (**Ref.** 4, p. 184)

359. **(A)** The eyes often close. Attacks are commonly precipitated by strong emotion, pleasurable or otherwise, especially by laughter, and the patient may be unable to move until he has controlled his emotions. (**Ref.** 4, p. 184)

360. **(C)** These are often vivid and frightening. Attacks occur while falling asleep. They are not uncommon in normal people, but may be especially vivid in narcoleptic patients. (**Ref.** 4, p. 185)

361. **(F)** The patient does not remember these episodes afterward. Sleepwalking occurs during stage IV NREM sleep, not during REM sleep. (**Ref.** 4, p. 185)

362. (E) Idiopathic narcolepsy, however, is not associated with any abnormal physical signs. The patient with symptomatic narcolepsy may show the signs of the causative lesion in the neighborhood of the pituitary and hypothalamus. (**Ref.** 4, pp. 183–184)

363. (D) The patient is rousable, but not normally alert and oriented when this is done. Parasomnia is commonly the result of a lesion involving the central reticular formation at the upper brain stem level. (**Ref.** 4, p. 183)

364. (B) Other external stimuli (eg, touch, noise, or music) may provoke an attack of reflex epilepsy. More recently, a further type of photoconvulsive epilepsy has been reported due to electronic video games. (**Ref.** 4, pp. 191–192)

365. (C) This may become bilateral when consciousness is usually lost. The EEG in simple motor epilepsy is likely to show a focal discharge. (**Ref.** 4, p. 190)

366. (A) In akinetic epilepsy, the only evidence for loss of consciousness is unawareness of the fall itself. Usually the patient can get up again at once. Cervical osteophytic compression of the vertebral arteries has been suggested as a possible factor in the production of ischemia. (**Ref.** 4, p. 192)

367. (E) There is generally a disturbance of the content of consciousness. Complex partial epilepsy may also produce the unconscious carrying out of some highly organized motor activity (eg, undressing). (**Ref.** 4, p. 191)

368. (F) There is transient weakness of the muscles involved in the convulsions. Jacksonian convulsions are usually associated with permanent weakness of the part of the body that is the focus of the fit, but after each convulsion there is often a temporary increase in both its severity and extent (Todd's paralysis). (**Ref.** 4, p. 232)

369. (D) This is rare; reportedly, it may continue for days or even months. It is the result of a focal lesion involving the corresponding area of the opposite motor cortex. (**Ref.** 4, pp. 192–193)

370. (B) This is inappropriate, unassociated with humor, and has occurred in psychomotor epilepsy. Complex partial seizures were formerly called "psychomotor disorders." **(Ref. 9, p. 2220)**

371. (A) EEG pattern is typical. Patients have mental retardation. There are multiple causes but in about half of the patients, no cause is found. **(Ref. 5, pp. 790–791)**

372. (A) This is also associated with developmental defects of the nervous system. Other metabolic causes include lipoidosis and pyridoxine deficiency. **(Ref. 5, p. 790)**

373. (A) However, the mental defect is not helped. Tonic spasms are frequently resistant to standard anticonvulsants. **(Ref. 5, p. 799)**

374. (C) Stroboscopic light has a similar effect. Both stimuli frequently precipitate or increase the incidence of bilateral paroxysmal discharges in seizure disorders characterized by primary engagement of bilateral structures. **(Ref. 5, p. 795)**

375. (E) Some feel that a limbic structural lesion is present in a high percentage of these cases. Complex partial seizures usually begin in the temporal lobe but may originate from the frontal, parietal, or occipital areas. **(Ref. 5, p. 786)**

376. (D) Defective TV sets have reportedly also caused this condition. Generalized clonicotonic seizures occur at some time in the course of epilepsy in most patients with seizures, regardless of the patient's usual clinical pattern. **(Ref. 5, pp. 787–788, 792)**

11

Neurologic Laboratory Procedures

DIRECTIONS (Questions 377–395): Each of the questions or incomplete statements below is followed by suggested answers or completions. Select the ONE that is BEST in each case.

---

377. In carpal tunnel syndrome

    A. only the median nerve motor conduction delay is found below the wrist

    B. both motor and sensory median nerve conduction delay are found below the wrist

    C. the sexes are affected approximately equally

    D. association with myxedema, arthritis, amyloid, and gout has been reported, but not acromegaly

    E. none of the above

378. To differentiate presenile dementia from intracranial tumor, one would employ
  A. calorics
  B. CT
  C. electroencephalography
  D. lumbar puncture
  E. routine skull x-rays

379. Abnormal values in lumbar CSF include
  A. 12 lymphocytes/mm
  B. 102 mg% protein
  C. 60 mg% glucose
  D. A and B but not C
  E. B and C but not A

380. The EEG
  A. frequency increases during the clonic phase of grand mal
  B. may be abnormal in 30% to 35% of the general population
  C. shows a 3/sec spike wave in petit mal epilepsy
  D. is normal in only 10% to 15% of awake adults with infrequent grand mal when a short record is taken
  E. none of the above

381. Among the activation techniques not used in electroencephalography is
  A. sleep
  B. convulsant drugs
  C. photic stimulation
  D. overhydration
  E. none of the above

382. The EEG is more helpful in tumors
  A. of the posterior fossa
  B. at the base of the brain
  C. of the cerebral hemispheres near the surface
  D. deep in the cerebrum
  E. none of the above

383. Nuclear magnetic resonance (NMR) or magnetic resonance imaging (MRI)
  A. is invaluable for emergency situations involving life support equipment
  B. helps evaluate patients who survive microsurgical treatment (with clipping) of an intracranial aneurysm
  C. is helpful in the follow-up of patients who have had metallic prostheses applied
  D. is limited primarily by the bony shadows of the posterior fossa
  E. shows plaques of multiple sclerosis better than does CT

384. The patient whose NMR (MRI) scan is shown (Figs. 11.1A and 11.1B)
  A. should be rushed to the operating room before it is too late
  B. has an intracerebral hemorrhage in a typical location
  C. has an intracerebral hemorrhage in an atypical location
  D. should have total tumor removal if possible; and subtotal resection is the next best procedure
  E. should have angiography to further delineate the abscess

Figure 11.1A.

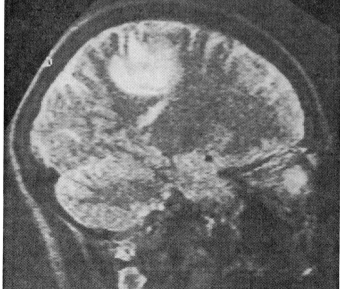

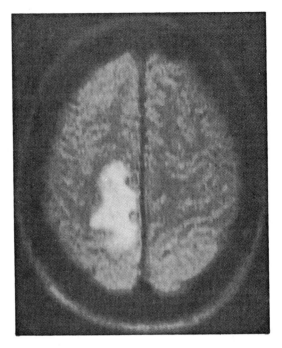

Figure 11.1B.

385. In the patient whose CT is shown (Fig. 11.2)
- **A.** duplication of the spinal cord may be expected
- **B.** spina bifida would be unusual
- **C.** symptoms beginning in adulthood would be unexpected
- **D.** of the various symptoms in this disorder, back pain would be one of the least likely to be present
- **E.** this acquired defect is seldom associated with congenital abnormalities of the CNS

386. Electromyography does not show
- **A.** signs of muscle denervation in neuropathic disorders such as amyotrophic lateral sclerosis
- **B.** little change in the number of muscle action potentials in myopathy
- **C.** a very characteristic repetitive pattern in myotonia
- **D.** reduction in the duration of potentials in myopathy
- **E.** none of the above

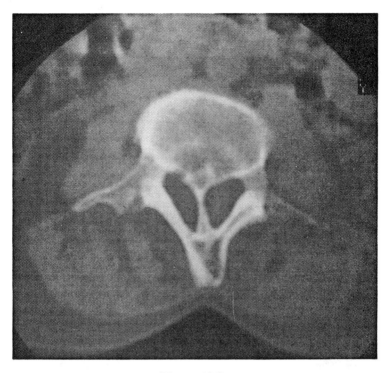

Figure 11.2.

387. Nerve conduction velocity measurement
    A. is useful only in the case of motor nerves
    B. is useful in many cases of neurologically asymptomatic diabetes mellitus
    C. shows slowing only in relatively few types of peripheral neuropathy
    D. if normal, rules out a nerve lesion
    E. none of the above

388. In the patient whose CT scan is shown (Fig. 11.3)
    A. right-sided hemisensory defects would be expected
    B. right-sided Foster Kennedy's syndrome would be expected
    C. right-sided incoordination would be expected
    D. papilledema and right homonymous hemianopsia would be expected
    E. none of the above

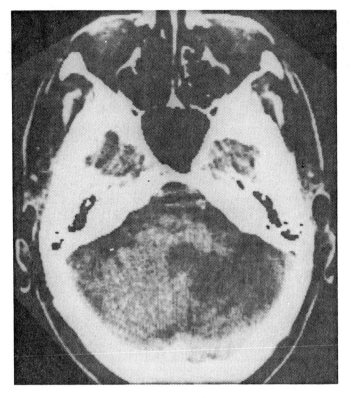

Figure 11.3.

389. This patient's CT lesion (Fig. 11.4) appeared the same with and without contrast. It is most likely
    A. cerebral infarction
    B. brain tumor
    C. cerebral hemorrhage
    D. aneurysm
    E. none of the above

390. This patient's CT lesion (Figs. 11.5A and 11.5B) showed slight enhancement with contrast injection. It is most likely
    A. cerebral infarction
    B. brain tumor
    C. cerebral hemorrhage
    D. aneurysm
    E. none of the above

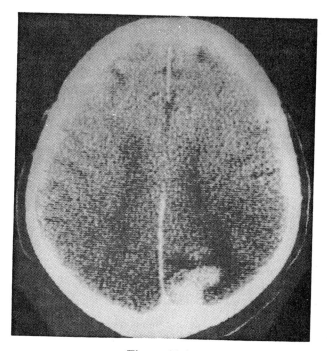

Figure 11.4.

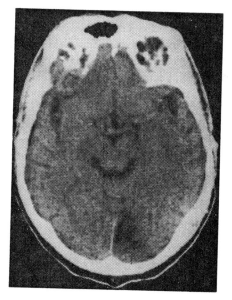

Figure 11.5A.

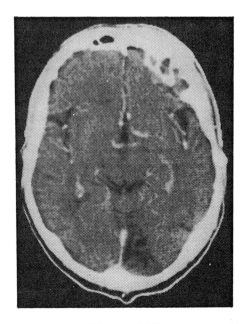

Figure 11.5B.

391. The accompanying angiogram (Fig. 11.6) illustrates a condition in which
   A. clipping of the neck is almost invariably performed
   B. early surgical treatment produces uniformly good results
   C. late surgical treatment produces uniformly good results
   D. no medical treatment has been reported to be helpful
   E. none of the above

392. The patient whose angiogram is shown (Fig. 11.7) had a subarachnoid hemorrhage. He
   A. has a posterior communicating artery aneurysm
   B. has a middle cerebral artery aneurysm
   C. has an anterior communicating artery aneurysm
   D. will die after a few weeks of recurrent hemorrhage unless microsurgical treatment is attempted

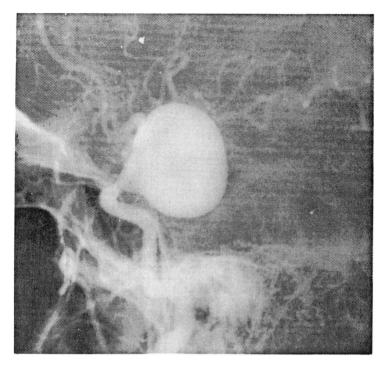

Figure 11.6.

    E. may survive the hemorrhage but will die of recurrent hemor-
        rhage in a few years unless microsurgical treatment is at-
        tempted

393. The patient whose CT scan is shown (Figs. 11.8A and 11.8B)
    A. must have burr holes, or death will occur
    B. can be treated successfully by medical therapy; sometimes
        steroids are used
    C. cannot show progressive resorption on serial CT scans
    D. must lead a restricted life
    E. none of the above

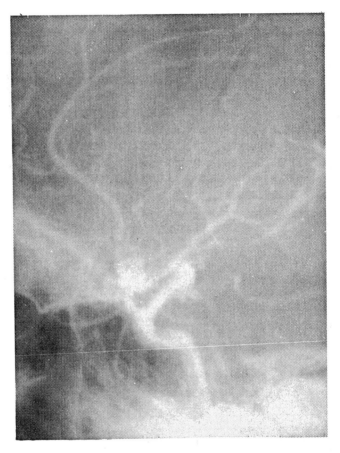

Figure 11.7.

394. In multiple sclerosis
   A. visual evoked potentials (VEP) are of no value
   B. nuclear magnetic resonance (NMR) is of no value because it is not capable of demonstrating necrotic or ischemic tissue
   C. positron emission tomography (PET) is routinely used in this country, with a miniature cyclotron and the injection of deoxyglucose containing radioactive fluorine
   D. digital vascular imaging (DVI) clearly shows abnormal circulatory patterns adjacent to the demyelinated areas
   E. none of the above

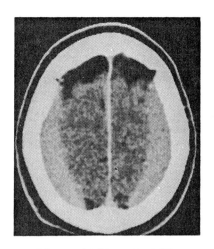

Figures 11.8A. and 11.8B.

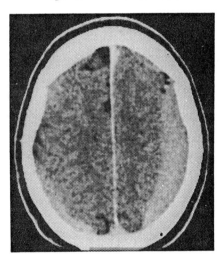

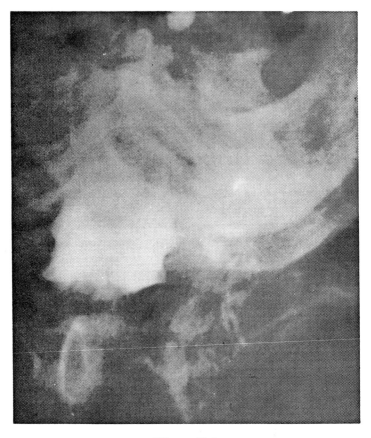

Figure 11.9.

395. In the patient whose myelogram is shown (Fig. 11.9)
- **A.** a sensory level would be unusual
- **B.** bilateral involvement of the lower extremities would be un-expected
- **C.** sphincter dysfunction would be most unusual
- **D.** vibration sense loss would be inappropriate
- **E.** none of the above

DIRECTIONS (Questions 396–405): The group of questions below consists of a list of lettered headings followed by a list of numbered words, phrases, or statements. For each numbered word, phrase, or statement, select the ONE lettered heading that is most closely associated with it. Each lettered heading may be selected once, more than once, or not at all.

Questions 396–405:

A. Produces osteomata, diffuse sclerosis of bone, and spicules protruding from the outer table
B. Extensive distribution of uniform-sized, destructive lesions
C. Normal sella, decalcified spine with compression fractures
D. Enlarged sella, sinuses, and mandible
E. Rare; destroys clivus
F. Monophasic and biphasic forms
G. Skull involvement may simulate metastases; most common in children
H. Parieto-occipital double lines of calcification, usually unilateral
I. Symmetric calcifications in the basal nuclei, especially the caudate, often the dentate
J. Suprasellar calcification in a young patient

396. Sturge-Weber disease

397. Hypoparathyroidism

398. Craniopharyngioma

399. Paget's disease

400. Leukemia

401. Chordoma

402. Chromophilic adenoma

403. Basophilic adenoma

404. Meningioma

405. Myeloma

DIRECTIONS (Questions 406–409): The set of lettered headings below is followed by a list of numbered words of phrases. For each numbered word or phrase select

    A. if the item is associated with A only
    B. if the item is associated with B only
    C. if the item is associated with both A and B
    D. if the item is associated with neither A nor B

Questions 406–409:

    A. Cervical spondylosis
    B. Amyotrophic lateral sclerosis
    C. Both
    D. Neither

406. Symptoms of cord damage tend to develop later, even if not present early

407. Long periods of nonprogressive disability are the rule

408. Bilateral extensor plantar responses

409. Cutaneous sensory loss in one or both lower extremities is frequent

---

DIRECTIONS (Questions 410–416): Each of the questions or incomplete statements below is followed by suggested answers or completions. Select the ONE that is BEST in each case.

---

410. The accompanying figure (Fig. 11.10) is a CT view of the head. On plain skull x-rays, this lesion
    A. would not be expected to show calcification within the mass
    B. would rarely exhibit hyperostosis

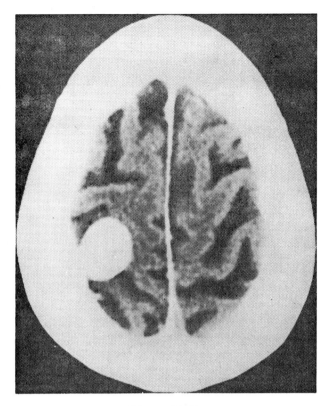

Figure 11.10.

    C. would frequently give evidence of its ability to invade the cortex

    D. would frequently show enlargement of the vascular channels over the vault of the skull

    E. would often give indication of its ability to invade the pia

411. In their common location, there is frequent involvement of the sagittal sinus and its cortical draining veins. Complete removal by operation

    A. is not difficult in the posterior fossa region

    B. is difficult in the parasagittal falx region

    C. is not difficult in the suprasella region

    D. is difficult in the convexity region

    E. is not difficult to remove in the primarily intraorbital region

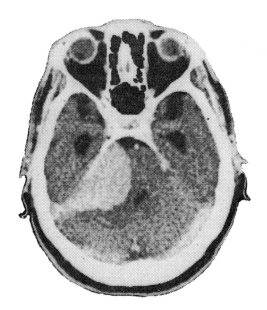

Figures 11.11A. and 11.11B.

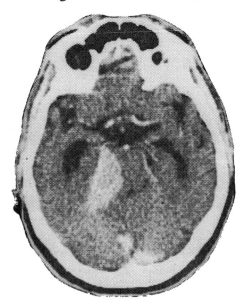

412. The accompanying figures (Figs. 11.11A and B) illustrate two views of the same problem. In lesions of this region

    A. one may expect cerebellar dysfunction but not occipital lobe dysfunction

    B. nystagmus may be prominent

    C. one may expect cerebellar dysfunction but not temporal lobe dysfunction

    D. vestibular response preservation is a non-specific finding as regards the different histologic types of neoplasm

    E. involvement of the clivus may produce cranial neuropathies but not myelopathy

413. Posterior fossa masses

    A. of the foramen magnum typically cause loss of light touch sensation (more prominent in the legs than in the arms)

    B. of the foramen magnum usually produce cranial neuropathies especially involving the ninth and tenth cranial nerves

    C. of the tentorium cause ipsilateral hemianopsia

    D. of the tentorium cause hydrocephalus

    E. arising from the petrous bone typically cause hydrocephalus without cranial neuropathies

414. In the condition illustrated by the accompanying figure (Fig. 11.12)

    A. although complications do occur after shunting, there have been no fatalities

    B. shunt complications include seizures but not subdural hematomas

    C. shunt complications include infections but not pulmonary embolism

    D. there is no consistent relationship between clinical improvement after shunting and reduction in ventricular size

    E. bilateral pyramidal and extrapyramidal signs are not part of this clinical picture

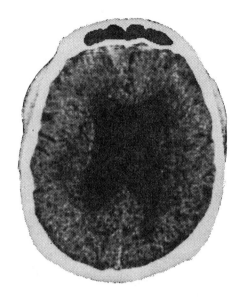

Figure 11.12.

415. In this condition
   A. radionuclide cisternography is generally accepted as the most accurate predictor of shunt success
   B. a callosal angle of less than 90 degrees on CT has been found to have prognostic value regarding surgery
   C. the presence of large lateral ventricles without visualization of the temporal horn tips indicates that the patient is a candidate for surgery
   D. metrizamide CT cisternography has shown promise as an additional predictor of shunt success
   E. clinical improvement after lumbar puncture has no predictive value regarding shunt success

416. In the condition illustrated by the accompanying figures (Figs. 11.13A and 11.13B)
   A. shunting appears to be indicated, at least from a radiographic standpoint

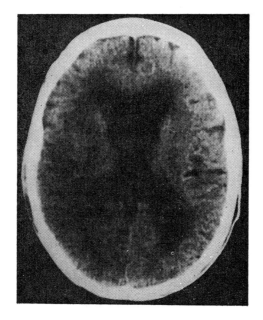

Figure 11.13A.

B. tricyclic treatment often helps
C. in a 41-year-old female this CT would be considered within normal limits
D. Pick's disease is not the first diagnostic choice
E. this plus one other laboratory test together can distinguish Alzheimer's disease from Pick's disease

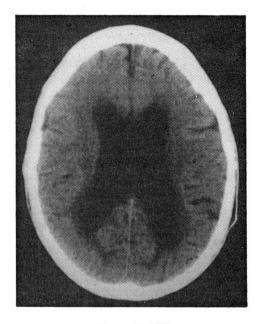

Figure 11.13B.

Answers and Discussion

377. (B) Most cases occur in middle-aged and often obese females. Treatment of an underlying systemic disease may be helpful; otherwise, steroid injections or surgery are used. However, postoperatively, sensory impairment, cutaneous hyperesthesia, and thenar muscle weakness may persist. (**Ref.** 9, pp. 2267–2268)

378. (B) CT scan and NMR (MRI) have now replaced PEG. NMR (MRI) involves no apparent hazard to the patient per se, and the results are often better than those obtained with CT. The patient should be screened for certain possible hazards (eg, pacemaker, prosthesis). (**Ref.** 4, pp. 156–159)

379. (D) CSF cell count reference range varies somewhat; some authors indicate not more than 3/mm^3. CSF protein reference range = 15–45 mg/dL; glucose reference range = 40–70 mg/dL. Microorganisms, parasites, and, rarely, tumor cells may also be found. A mononuclear pleocytosis is the most frequent reaction to infections with neurotropic viruses, though polymorphonuclear cells are sometimes present in such cases when the infection is most acute. (**Ref.** 4, p. 151; **Ref.** 9, pp. 2397, 2399)

380. (C) Ten percent of normal and healthy individuals have an EEG which is electrically "abnormal." A focal abnormality does not necessarily mean that the area is the site of the original discharge. Some apparent focal discharges may not originate in the cortex because stimulation of subcortical structures in animals can result in surface EEG spikes and other pathophysiologic responses.

During a seizure, spikes of low voltage gradually increase in amplitude and decrease in frequency. (**Ref.** 5, p. 795; **Ref.** 4, p. 155)

381. **(E)** The main use is in the activation of a focal abnormality. Hyperventilation and sleep deprivation are also frequently used. (**Ref.** 5, p. 794)

382. **(C)** Deep tumors or posterior fossa tumors may be accompanied by diffuse slowing of electrical activity. Focal abnormalities in electrical activity are helpful in indicating the site of a lesion. Their character does not make possible an absolute differential diagnosis between a tumor and other lesions of the cortex. (**Ref.** 5, p. 280)

383. **(E)** It is also superior to CT scans in demonstrating post-traumatic contusions and intraaxial brain stem tumors. The technique is totally noninvasive and free of exposure to x-rays. The presence of metallic structures (eg, life support systems, clips, or prostheses), often contraindicate the use of MRI. (**Ref.** 9, pp. 84–86, 2058–2059)

384. **(C)** This is a relatively unusual location for intracerebral hemorrhage and raises the question of relatively unusual etiologies in the latter's causation—especially since this particular patient had no obvious risk factors (eg, relatively young age, no known systemic medical illnesses such as hypertension, diabetes, or blood dyscrasia). The patient recovered with careful clinical neurologic monitoring and no operation. Repeat NMR confirmed shrinkage of the hemorrhage. (**Ref.** 5, pp. 185–186)

385. **(A)** This bony abnormality divides the spinal canal, leading to duplication of the spinal cord. There is usually evidence of spina bifida on plain films. Patients developing symptoms in adulthood almost always have some cutaneous abnormality, especially hypertrichosis over the sacral area. This condition may also be associated with other CNS abnormalities. (**Ref.** 9, p. 2258)

386. **(E)** The EMG is most useful in diagnosing disease of the motor unit (ie, ventral horn cell, central nerve root, motor nerve, myoneural junction and muscle). It is also helpful in differentiating

demyelinating neuropathy from axonal neuropathy. (**Ref. 9, pp. 2056–2058**)

387. (B) Slowing of conduction is observed in many kinds of peripheral neuropathy; sensory neuropathy may also produce slowing of conduction. Measurement of the F response is used; this involves analyzing antidromic and orthodromic stimulations. Measurement of the H reflex consists of utilizing the electrical equivalent of the stretch reflex. (**Ref. 9, pp. 2056–2058**)

388. (C) This is a large right cerebellar infarction. The lateral lobes of the cerebellum are concerned chiefly with movements of the limbs on the same side of the body and of the eyes to that side, while the vermis is concerned chiefly with what may be termed "axial functions," namely, speech, the maintenance of the upright posture of the trunk, standing, and walking. (**Ref. 4, p. 106**)

389. (C) The patient was elderly and hypertensive; no additional cerebral vascular abnormality was seen. Arteriolar microaneurysm rupture is felt to be the most common cause. CT is helpful in separating the clinically inobvious hemorrhage from infarction. After 48 hours, MR (= MRI) is more sensitive to blood than CT. (**Ref. 5, pp. 217–220; Ref. 9, p. 2059**)

390. (A) Small cystic infarctions or lacunes are the most common forms of infarction. This patient has a somewhat larger left occipital infarction. After cerebral infarction, contrast CT shows about half of the supratentorial infarctions on the day of ictus and about three-quarters of them about 10 days after onset. (**Ref. 5, pp. 193–194**)

391. (E) Because of frequently poor microsurgical results in giant aneurysms, carotid ligation is still attempted, despite its ability (as in the actual case shown) to provoke fatal aneurysm rupture in a previously unruptured aneurysm. Results with a very small number of such patients treated with medical-hypotensive therapy and followed now, in some cases for more than 10 years, appear to be encouraging. Articles on surgical treatment (of this less common type of aneurysm problem) are published from time to time, but overall, treatment of these symptomatic, though unruptured, giant aneurysms remains controversial. (**Ref.** 7, pp. 207–218)

392. (C) The patient remained well into his early eighties, with normal mental status, and, in fact, had climbed six flights of stairs at age 81 without significant difficulty. He died one month before his 84th birthday of an unrelated illness (chest carcinoma; the patient had been a heavy smoker for years). He had been followed for almost 27 years since his hemorrhage, which was treated with medical-hypotensive therapy only; the aneurysm never rebled. Excellent long-term follow-up results in patients with ruptured brain aneurysm, treated entirely medically with hypotension, are now routinely found. (**Ref.** 15, pp. 1357–1361; **Ref.** 16, pp. 7–8; **Ref.** 18, p. I-145)

393. (B) In one series of more than 100 patients with subdural hematomas, it was shown that in most instances, surgical treatment is completely unnecessary because the patients can be treated medically with excellent results, such as the patient whose bilateral subdural hematomas are shown. Medical treatment requires adequate neurologic facilities. This is mandatory. The point here is that while surgical treatment is the older and most popular approach, a very effective alternative method of medical treatment has become available. It should also be added here that another previously very popular surgical treatment (extracranial-intracranial anastomosis) for another kind of cerebrovascular disorder (occlusive cerebrovascular disease) has recently been discredited, to the surprise of some, by a very large randomized study. (**Ref.** 8, pp. 1869–1871)

394. (E) VEP are of value and NMR(MR) can be confirmatory. PET is hampered by the need for a nearby cyclotron; Japan has developed a miniature cyclotron, the use of which is being evaluated. (**Ref.** 5, p. 754; **Ref.** 9, p. 7060)

395. (E) If the tumor is laterally placed, Brown-Séquard's syndrome may occur. Usually the syndrome is incomplete. (**Ref.** 5, p. 351)

396. (H) In encephalotrigeminal angiomatosis, calcium is deposited in the cortex; cortical atrophy is usually present. In this condition, a facial nevus is associated with seizures, hemiplegia, retardation, and glaucoma. (**Ref.** 5, pp. 582–584)

397. (I) This is also found in pseudohypoparathyroidism or in the absence of any recognizable cause. The calcifications may be seen on plain radiographs of the skull; they are visualized in greater detail via CT. (**Ref.** 5, p. 833)

398. (J) A very high percentage of these tumors show calcification. Although the sella turcica may be eroded, it is uncommon for it to be ballooned, as in pituitary adenomas. (**Ref.** 5, pp. 326–328)

399. (F) The monophasic form (which is destructive only) eventually progresses to the more common biphasic form. Radiographically, one sees an enormous skull with "cotton wool" appearance of the bones of the vault. In advanced cases, platybasia may be present. (**Ref.** 5, pp. 863–864)

400. (G) Punctate areas of rarefaction are found; occasionally, new bone formation occurs. CT may show hydrocephalus, subarachnoid enhancement, and intracerebral hemorrhages. (**Ref.** 5, p. 851)

401. (E) With growth, adjacent posterior and middle fossa bone is destroyed. The bony erosion may be seen on plain skull radiographs or on CT scans. This tumor also occurs, in the sacrococcygeal region, and a smaller number occur elsewhere along the spine. (**Ref.** 5, p. 328)

402. (D) The sella is usually not as enlarged as it is in chromophobe adenoma; the calvarium is thickened. A more satisfactory classification divides pituitary tumors into secreting and non-secreting types. CT visualizes the lesions especially well with contrast material. MRI is even more sensitive. (**Ref.** 5, pp. 318–325; **Ref.** 9, p. 2234)

403. (C) This tumor is rare; it causes diffuse skeletal osteoporosis, especially of the thoracic spine. Basophilic adenomas of the pituitary associated with bilateral adrenocortical hyperplasia and the features of hypercortisonism constitute a disorder first described by Cushing. (**Ref.** 9, p. 1304)

404. (A) Plain skull films often suggest the diagnosis and an isotopic brain scan frequently visualizes the lesion but CT and MRI are the most definitive procedures. (**Ref.** 5, pp. 292–293)

405. (B) The lesions are entirely destructive; there is no evidence of bone proliferation. Characteristic multiple osteolytic lesions are seen on radiographs of the skull and other bones. The cord may be compromised by a pathologic vertebral fracture. (**Ref.** 5, pp. 852–853)

406. (B) Terminally, there is widespread motor cell involvement. However, there is no specific diagnostic test for amyotrophic lateral sclerosis. (**Ref.** 5, pp. 409–411)

407. (A) The course varies considerably. In patients not treated surgically, the condition sometimes becomes arrested or even improves spontaneously. Amyotrophic lateral sclerosis is a progressive disease, although there are cases of long duration; those generally have few if any upper motor neuron signs and may be more accurately regarded as spinal muscular atrophy. (**Ref.** 5, pp. 361, 409–411)

408. (C) These two diseases may coexist. One of the diagnostic problems involves the possible coexistence of cervical spondylosis with any of several other spinal cord diseases because the former is so commonly found in the general population. (**Ref.** 5, pp. 409–411)

409. (D) Sensory loss is not a feature of amyotrophic lateral sclerosis. Vibration sense impairment in the lower extremities is not unusual in cervical spondylosis. Infrequently, a sensory level is found and is helpful diagnostically. (**Ref.** 5, pp. 409–411)

410. (D) Despite the widespread use of CT, careful evaluation of the plain skull radiograph is still helpful. In this case, headaches, originally attributed by others to the tumor, decreased when the dosage of vasodilator medication (for the patient's cardiac disease) was reduced. An operation was felt to be unnecessary. She has been followed for more than 10 years with periodic clinical neurologic assessment and occasional repeat CT scans. (**Ref.** 5, pp. 291–297)

411. (B) Recurrence of tumor after apparently successful surgery is not unusual; it may take a few years or many years. (**Ref. 5, pp. 291–297**)

412. (B) Meningiomas in the cerebellopontine angle produce a syndrome similar to that of an acoustic neurinoma. Surgery can damage cranial nerves as well as vertebral arteries. Clivus involvement can cause high spinal cord dysfunction. (**Ref. 5, pp. 291–297**)

413. (D) Foramen magnum tumors cause loss of light touch more prominently in the arms than in the legs. The twelfth and eleventh cranial nerves are more often involved. Tentorial lesions cause contralateral hemianopsia. (**Ref. 5, pp. 296–297, 355**)

414. (D) In one report, the complication rate was 44%. Despite the name ("normal pressure hydrocephalus"), intermittent intracranial hypertension has been reported while monitoring suspected cases. (**Ref. 5, pp. 255–262**)

415. (D) Despite replacement of PEG by CT and MRI, plus some replacement of radionuclide CSF studies by CT metrizamide cisternography, accurate selection of patients for shunting remains elusive. Even under the best circumstances, it has been reported that a complication rate of 35% is not uncommon. (**Ref. 5, p. 262; Ref. 9, pp. 2235–2237**)

416. (D) This patient has diffuse atrophy. In addition, even if focal atrophy alone were demonstrable, this may also occur in Alzheimer's disease. (**Ref. 5, pp. 637–643; Ref. 9, pp. 2090–2091**)

12

Phenomenology and Anatomy

DIRECTIONS (Questions 417–460): Each of the questions or incomplete statements below is followed by suggested answers or completions. Select the ONE that is BEST in each case.

---

417. In Ondine's curse, respiration
   A. is variably irregular in rate and amplitude
   B. on a voluntary basis is preserved, but automatic respiration is lost
   C. consists of inspiratory pauses and is seen in pantine lesions
   D. consists of periods of hyperventilation alternating with periods of apnea in a crescendo-decrescendo fashion
   E. consists of cluster breathing with less smooth waxing and waning

418. In cases of non-right-handedness (left-handedness or various degrees of ambidexterity) with language disorder, the lesion is
  A.   more commonly in the left hemisphere
  B.   more commonly in the right hemisphere
  C.   just as likely to be in one hemisphere as in the other
  D.   almost invariably in the left hemisphere
  E.   almost invariably in the right hemisphere

419. Causes of mutism usually do not include
  A.   uncooperativeness
  B.   depression or schizophrenia
  C.   diffuse brain dysfunction such as subarachnoid hemorrhage, trauma, or metabolic disorders
  D.   mid-brain, pontine, or bilateral cranial nerve lesions
  E.   aphasia

420. The patient who requests a "pin-pink" instead of a "pen" is exhibiting
  A.   literal or phonemic paraphasia
  B.   verbal paraphasia
  C.   Gerstmann's syndrome
  D.   anosognosia
  E.   a typical callosal syndrome

421. In Gerstmann's syndrome, the patient will
  A.   carry out verbal commands with the right hand
  B.   not carry out verbal commands with the left hand
  C.   name (concealed) objects held in the right hand
  D.   not name (concealed) objects held in the left hand but with the left hand; can draw that object previously held in it
  E.   none of the above

422. In denial of illness
  A.   when the disability is admitted, the patient generally is quite concerned
  B.   the patient usually has a right hemiplegia
  C.   the situation is, unfortunately, generally permanent
  D.   the lesion is usually in the right hemisphere
  E.   the lesion is usually in the left hemisphere

423. In apraxia, the defect is generally
- **A.** least marked to verbal commands
- **B.** most marked on imitation of the examiner
- **C.** less marked in the handling of objects
- **D.** equal for all these
- **E.** none of the above

424. In typical organic causes of "amnesia"
- **A.** the patient may have a very selective form of memory disorder (eg, denying that he is married)
- **B.** the patient may have a total or global form of memory disorder, usually persisting for days, except for retrograde amnesia, which may last for weeks
- **C.** the patient, who is not aphasic, is unable to state his own name
- **D.** fugue states occur and may affect the patient's reporting of memory involving several weeks
- **E.** none of the above

425. In memory disorders
- **A.** the hippocampus and mammillary bodies probably play minor roles
- **B.** short-term memory probably involves a molecular change
- **C.** the limbic system is probably most important
- **D.** long-term storage probably involves continuation of nervous activity
- **E.** none of the above

426. In Korsakoff's syndrome
- **A.** thiamine deficiency may cause severe lesions in the mammillary bodies
- **B.** the hippocampus is more markedly involved than the dorsal medial nuclei of the thalamus
- **C.** memory disorder is less prominent than other intellectual features
- **D.** profound recent and remote memory loss are noted, along with confabulation
- **E.** none of the above

427. In testing for dementia
   A. the antecedent intellectual development plays little role
   B. a patient with Korsakoff's syndrome will be expected to have difficulty naming objects but will know where he is
   C. constructional capacity and proverb definition are not really relevant
   D. recent memory and attention are among the least useful
   E. none of the above

428. In the differential diagnosis of dementia
   A. it is important to look for spastic weakness of one side and contralateral loss of pain and temperature sensation
   B. symptom development, neurologic signs, and laboratory results are helpful in pointing to specific pathology
   C. reversible and irreversible pathologies tend to produce different symptomatology
   D. vitamin deficiencies and endocrinopathy are unimportant
   E. none of the above

429. Examples of referred pain do not include
   A. toothache pain noted in the temporomandibular region
   B. subdiaphragmatic abscess producing ipsilateral posterior shoulder pain
   C. mid-esophageal pain felt substernally
   D. angina pectoris pain felt by the medial aspect of the arm
   E. none of the above

430. Examples of truncal referred pain do not include
   A. pain originating at the lower third of the esophagus and stomach referred to the epigastric area
   B. duodenal ulcer pain referred to the epigastrium
   C. appendiceal pain referred to the hypogastrium
   D. angina pectoris pain felt at the jaw
   E. none of the above

431. In genitourinary referred pain
   A. testicular pain is referred to the perineum
   B. urethral pain is referred to the flank
   C. ureteral colic produces pain along the rectus abdominus, then into the flank and groin

D. the pain is felt in the flank only

E. the pain is felt in the groin only

432. A patient with a parietal lesion might be expected to demonstrate

    A. visual inattention but normal opticokinetic nystagmus

    B. Gerstmann's syndrome in anterior lesions

    C. impaired position sense; intact stereognosis

    D. impaired two-point discrimination and a visual field cut

    E. none of the above

433. Postherpetic neuralgia

    A. when treated surgically, yields uncertain results

    B. almost invariably subsides after four to five days

    C. is treated by terry cloth towel massage in order to decrease the sensory input

    D. does not respond to transcutaneous nerve stimulation

    E. should not be treated with psychotrophic drugs

434. In intractable pain

    A. bilateral frontal lobotomy or cingulotomy should be tried because they seldom disturb the patient's personality

    B. some of the most difficult situations occur when the pain fulfills an emotional need

    C. metastatic disease may require limbic surgery in order to modify the perception of pain more than the reaction to it

    D. dorsal column stimulation is being used increasingly often

    E. acupuncture's effect is not reversed by naloxone

435. Pain-sensitive structures of the head do not include

    A. all extracranial tissues, especially the arteries

    B. the large venous sinuses and their surface venous tributaries, some basal dura and basal arteries

    C. fifth, seventh, ninth, and tenth cranial nerves

    D. the first three cervical nerves

    E. none of the above

436. Headache has been said to be due primarily to intracranial arterial dilatation and distention in the case of
- **A.** nitrite administration
- **B.** carbon dioxide inhalation
- **C.** meningitis
- **D.** lumbar puncture
- **E.** fever but not hypoxia

437. Postlumbar puncture headache
- **A.** characteristically develops in the frontal region
- **B.** can often be avoided by using a small needle
- **C.** is often temporally aggravated by attempted "replacement" with saline
- **D.** can usually be prevented by keeping the patient recumbent after the procedure
- **E.** none of the above

438. Extracranially caused headache is due primarily to
- **A.** cranial artery dilatation and distention, plus the major craniofacial neuralgias
- **B.** cranial artery dilatation and distention, plus sustained contraction of face, scalp, and neck skeletal muscles
- **C.** cranial artery dilatation and distention, plus nonspecific cranial artery inflammation
- **D.** sustained skeletal muscle contraction (face, scalp, and neck), plus pain secondary to diseased nasal, eye, and dental tissues
- **E.** trauma, infection, or new growth of extracranial tissues

439. In cluster headache
- **A.** ipsilateral Horner's syndrome may be present
- **B.** alcohol may induce attacks either during or between cluster periods
- **C.** the attacks typically last for 8 to 10 hours and then subside
- **D.** the pain is usually bilateral
- **E.** women are affected more often than men

440. In migraine
   - **A.** during attacks, there is a decreased urinary excretion of serotonin metabolites
   - **B.** reserpine may produce a rise in the level of serum serotonin; it also may induce a migraine attack
   - **C.** serotonin has been said to compete with administered methysergide for receptor sites in pain-sensitive vessels
   - **D.** during attacks, platelet monoamine oxidase activity rises
   - **E.** decreased platelet aggregability has been noted

441. In headaches presumed to be due to contraction of skeletal muscle
   - **A.** amitriptyline is not effective
   - **B.** the headache may last for days, with an occasional maximum of two to three weeks
   - **C.** there is commonly tenderness to palpation, and even combing the hair causes pain
   - **D.** heat aggravates the pain
   - **E.** the pain is invariably bilateral

442. In otherwise completely well and symptom-free patients with arterial hypertension
   - **A.** 50% to 60% have been found to have frequent severe headaches
   - **B.** the extent of the blood pressure elevation correlates with the severity of the attacks
   - **C.** daily fluctuations in the elevation of blood pressure correlate well with the occurrence of the headaches
   - **D.** headaches tend to occur at the end of the day
   - **E.** none of the above

443. In extracranial headache due to dental disease
   - **A.** distant tissues may show hyperalgesia, and tenderness, but not vasomotor reactions
   - **B.** tenderness and pain in the neck and shoulders have been reported
   - **C.** eyeball tenderness does not occur
   - **D.** reddening of the conjunctivae does not occur
   - **E.** occipital pain does not occur

444. Pain in the ear does not occur in
  A. herpes zoster of the fifth and seventh cranial nerves; rarely in the ninth cranial nerve
  B. glossopharyngeal neuralgia
  C. dental disease, acute tonsillitis, and inflammatory disease of the posterior fossa
  D. laryngeal tumors
  E. none of the above

445. In sensorineural hearing loss
  A. the Rinne test is normal
  B. recruitment is absent in cochlear dysfunction but present in nerve disease
  C. tone decay is present in cochlear disorders but absent in nerve lesions
  D. diplacusis is absent
  E. patients prefer loud speech

446. In conductive hearing loss
  A. complete failure of inner ear development may be causative
  B. cochleosaccular dysgenesis is the most common cause
  C. temporal bone laminagrams may be useful diagnostically
  D. impacted cerumen plays no role
  E. suppurative but not serous otitis impairs conduction of air-borne sound

447. In virus-associated hearing deficits
  A. mumps causes bilateral deafness, with occasional vestibular dysfunction
  B. "cochleitis" may be due to inflammatory but not vascular disorders
  C. Ramsey-Hunt syndrome does not occur
  D. adults may suffer sudden unilateral hearing loss
  E. none of the above

448. In otologic syphilis
  A. eventual total deafness is uncommon; sudden total deafness in one ear does occur
  B. fluctuating progressive sensorineural hearing loss and vertigo are found

C. recurrent interstitial keratitis but not Clutton's joints is found

D. there is no evidence that long-term cortisone treatment is of value in any of the manifestations of congenital syphilis

E. deafness is part of the syndrome of early congenital lues

449. Otosclerosis

A. is common and usually inherited as a recessive trait

B. is due to an overgrowth of labyrinthine capsular bone, which produces fixation of the malleus and stapes

C. has been treated by horizontal canal fenestration, stapes mobilization, and stapedectomy with replacement

D. produces noticeable hearing loss, in most cases, as early as ages 40 to 50

E. none of the above

450. In the Argyll-Robertson pupil

A. mydriasis is present

B. reaction to mydriatics is prompt

C. reaction to light is prompt

D. reaction to convergence is prompt

E. none of the above

451. In the tonic pupil

A. the abnormality is usually bilateral

B. mydriasis is present

C. reaction to light is prompt

D. reaction to convergence is prompt

E. the deep tendon reflexes are usually hyperactive

452. If both jaw jerk and arm jerk are very exaggerated, the lesion is usually

A. just below the foramen magnum

B. at the foramen magnum

C. in the medulla

D. below the pons

E. above the pons

453. An upper motor neuron lesion of the hypoglossal fibers
A. may cause some contralateral loss of function
B. is asymptomatic
C. causes marked deviation of the protruded tongue to the side of the lesion
D. is generally followed by fasciculations
E. leads to atrophy

454. Deafness
A. when bilateral, is invariably peripheral in origin
B. is generally unilateral in central lesions
C. occurs in fractures but not in tumors at the base of the brain
D. does not occur in congenital lues
E. may be preceded by years of tinnitus

455. If tapping the pes anserinus causes bilateral twitching of the facial muscles, one would expect
A. meningitis
B. hypoglossal lesions
C. pseudobulbar palsy
D. tetany
E. hysteria

456. If a supine patient tries to raise one leg and the pressure on the bed of the contralateral heel does not increase, one would suspect
A. tabes dorsalis
B. myasthenia gravis
C. thoracic cord tumor
D. hysteria
E. normal findings

457. In the differential diagnosis of trigeminal neuralgia, it should be remembered that
A. hypalgesic areas within the distribution of the fifth cranial nerve are found in one-third to one-half of the cases
B. the corneal reflex is preserved, and there is no basic abnormality in motor function
C. eating is unaffected as a rule
D. the pain may be a symptom of Gasserian ganglion tumor but not of multiple sclerosis
E. the pain occurs frequently at night

458. In glossopharyngeal neuralgia
   A. the trigger zone is in the posterior pharynx but not in the tonsillar fossa
   B. syncope has been reported due to severe bradycardia and even arrest
   C. the patient's description of the sensation of pain does not resemble that of tic douloureux
   D. tonsillar tumor pain does not mimic this
   E. carbamazepine is ineffective

459. In tabetic pain
   A. the patient generally gives a history of pain in the trunk or upper extremities
   B. the pain is frequently described as paroxysmal
   C. spirochetes can be demonstrated in the dorsal root ganglia or posterior columns
   D. carbamazepine is ineffective
   E. surgery is effective

460. In causalgia the
   A. condition follows a partial injury to peripheral nerves, especially the sciatic or radial nerve
   B. pain is almost continuous and usually is burning in nature
   C. involved extremity is cool and hairless; the skin is shiny and smooth; atrophy does not occur
   D. sympathetic block is of no value
   E. lidocaine is of no value

DIRECTIONS (Questions 461–464): Each set of lettered headings below is followed by a list of numbered words or phrases. For each numbered word or phrase select

  A. if the item is associated with A only
  B. if the item is associated with B only
  C. if the item is associated with both A and B
  D. if the item is associated with neither A nor B

Questions 461–464:

  A. Benign essential tremor
  B. Parkinsonian tremor
  C. Both
  D. Neither

461. Typically involves the upper limbs and head

462. A strong family history is generally noted

463. Propranolol effective

464. Onset usually in adult life

DIRECTIONS (Questions 465–493): Each group of questions below consists of lettered headings followed by a list of numbered words or statements. For each numbered word or statement, select the ONE lettered heading that is most closely associated with it. Each lettered heading may be selected once, more than once, or not at all.

Questions 465–467:

  A. Feeling that one's ear is "ballooning out six inches or more"
  B. Feeling that "I was going fast" and "as if everyone was talking too fast and moving too fast"
  C. Feeling that "I was very tall—able to look down on the tops of others' heads"

465. Epilepsy

466. Migraine

467. Viral encephalitis

Questions 468–470:

    A. Creutzfeldt-Jakob disease
    B. Familial or sporadic essential myoclonus
    C. Palatal myoclonus

468. Benign myoclonic jerks

469. Symptomatic myoclonus

470. Rhythmic myoclonus

Questions 471–473:

    A. Ocular myoclonus
    B. Levodopa, tricyclics
    C. Associated with petit mal or grand mal seizures

471. Symptomatic myoclonus

472. Benign myoclonic jerks

473. Rhythmic myoclonus

Questions 474–478:

    A. Fluent; abundant; (–) comprehension; (–) repetition
    B. Fluent; (+) comprehension; (–) repetition
    C. (+) repetition
    D. Nonfluent; effortful; (+) comprehension; (–) repetition
    E. Nonfluent; scant; (–) comprehension; (–) repetition

474. Broca aphasia

475. Wernicke aphasia

476. Conduction aphasia

477. Global aphasia

478. Transcortical motor or transcortical sensory aphasia

Questions 479–483:

    A. Autosomal dominant with close to complete penetrance; depression or schizophreniform behavior common

    B. Typically progresses in steps with minor or major worsening, occasionally with some improvement between episodes; prominent motor changes; imaging studies helpful

    C. Early appearance and rapid progression over several months of seizures of upper motor neuron dysfunction plus increasing dementia and prominent EEG changes

    D. Insidious onset; progressive; associated with broad based ataxia and urinary incontinence; often with history of remote subarachnoid hemorrhage, recurrent head trauma, or meningeal infection

    E. Failure of recent memory; emotional behavior disturbances; sparing of primary motor and sensory functions

479. Hydrocephalic dementia

480. Huntington's disease

481. Creutzfeldt-Jakob disease

482. Multi-infarct dementia

483. Alzheimer's disease

Questions 484–488:

    A. Dancing, the playing of instruments, typing, or swimming

    B. Materials improperly learned or not learned at all

    C. As short as hours or days (eg, post-traumatic); or years or even decades (eg, Korsakoff's syndrome)

    D. Factual knowledge

    E. Digit span testing or other material held for less than 60 seconds; spared in most amnesias

484. Declarative memory

485. Procedural memory

486. Immediate or short-term memory

487. Retrograde amnesia

488. Anterograde amnesia

Questions 489–493:

    A. Patients are distressed by it and ask repeatedly where they are and what is going on; patient can identify himself
    B. Severe amnesia including both anterograde and retrograde memories with lack of insight and confabulation
    C. Severe anterograde amnesia with largely spared retrograde memory, generic memories, and procedural learning
    D. Episodes in which patients are generally noninquisitive and inattentive
    E. Episodes may include disorientation to self; communication often reduced to monosyllables

489. Surgery (bilateral medial temporal globe resection) for epilepsy

490. Psychogenic amnesia

491. Korsakoff's syndrome

492. Transient global amnesia

493. Status epilepticus with partial complex or petit mal seizures

Answers and Discussion

417. (B) This is said to be due to medullary lesions. As the patient becomes less alert, apnea may be fatal. Other ominous respiratory signs are end-respiratory pushing and "fish mouthing" (ie, lower jaw depression with inspiration). **(Ref. 5, pp. 22–23)**

418. (A) The non-right-handedness situation is more complex, but it has been suggested that the lesion is still more likely to be in the left hemisphere than in the right. **(Ref. 9, pp. 2085–2087)**

419. (E) Even severe aphasics are usually not mute. This term is applied to complete loss of speech in a conscious patient in the absence of both aphasia and anarthria; it is usually but not always due to a psychologic cause. **(Ref. 4, p. 133)**

420. (A) The sound is well articulated but incorrect. In verbal paraphasias, words are replaced by others that have a similar meaning. Wernicke's aphasia is considered sensory aphasia and Broca's aphasia is considered motor or sensory. In Broca's aphasia, there may be an associated right hemiparesis. **(Ref. 5, pp. 10–11)**

421. (E) The description is that of a callosal syndrome. Gerstmann's syndrome includes finger agnosia, agraphia, acalculia, and a failure to discriminate between right and left. **(Ref. 4, pp. 140–142)**

422. (D) Although not all patients with denial of illness have right hemisphere disease, it is frequently a striking feature and can affect management. Statements regarding precise localization of the lesion are of doubtful validity. **(Ref. 9, pp. 2081–2082)**

423. (E) The patient is unable to perform a learned act in response to a stimulus that would normally elicit it; there is no weakness, incoordination, or other deficit to account for it. Apraxic disorders are broadly considered to be the body movement equivalents of the dysphasias. (**Ref.** 5, p. 12)

424. (E) Temporal lobe epilepsy may produce some fugue states, but these are generally brief. In organic memory loss, disorientation occurs for time and place but not for self. (**Ref.** 9, pp. 2083–2085, 2239–2240; **Ref.** 4, p. 277)

425. (C) Unilateral damage to the human hippocampus produces relatively subtle defects, whereas bilateral damage is devastating and causes profound and usually permanent deficits in intermediate memory affecting especially the verbal-visual-spatial spheres. (**Ref.** 9, pp. 2083–2084; **Ref.** 4, pp. 354–355)

426. (D) Mammillary-hippocampal lesions must be bilateral if the memory deficit is to be permanent. The memory failure in thiamine deficiency is accompanied consistently by bilateral damage to the dorsal medial nucleus of the thalamus. In Western countries, nutritional Korsakoff's syndrome most frequently affects alcoholics. (**Ref.** 9, p. 2084)

427. (E) This refers to a generalized deterioration in intellectual capacity rather than a loss of more specific functions such as language (in aphasia) and memory (in Korsakoff's syndrome). In the progressive dementias, families or work associates generally notice a change before the patient does. (**Ref.** 9, pp. 2087–2088)

428. (B) Symptoms of dementia are not pathology specific. Certain laboratory tests must be done so as not to overlook a treatable cause (eg, vitamin deficiencies and endocrinopathy). (**Ref.** 9, pp. 2089–2090)

429. (E) Referred pain may occur with or without awareness of the primary site. Usually but not always, it is cutaneous and is evoked by disease of deep structures innervated by the same dermatome. (**Ref.** 9, pp. 106, 2249–2250)

430. (E) Pain is referred from the lower esophagus, stomach, and small intestine to the epigastrium; and from the large bowel to the hypogastrium. Sometimes pain is referred at a greater distance from the primary site to segments not similarly innervated, and there the mechanism is perplexing (eg, anginal pain referred to the jaw). (**Ref.** 9, pp. 106, 2249–2250)

431. (C) GU pain is referred to the hypogastric area and the flank. Theories suggested to account for referred pain include division of the same nerve into deep and superficial branches, release of chemical mediators in the nervous system, and convergence of cutaneous and visceral nerves into common synaptic pools at the spinal cord. (**Ref.** 9, pp. 2249–2250)

432. (D) Visual inattention may be present. Pursuit eye movements and stereognosis may be impaired. Pain appears to be consciously perceived in the upper brainstem and the thalamus; its localization and recognition of the stimulus for it depend upon thalamoparietal projections. Sensory deficits that are not apparent on single stimulation may be brought out by double simultaneous stimulation. (**Ref.** 9, pp. 2081–2082, 2128–2129)

433. (A) This condition frequently presents a difficult management problem, thereby giving rise to a variety of therapeutic approaches. Carbamazepine is the drug of choice for postherpetic neuralgia but may be more effective when combined with other tricyclic compounds. (**Ref.** 9, p. 2197; **Ref.** 5, pp. 117–118)

434. (B) The decision regarding therapy depends upon the life expectancy, as well as the pain's intensity and the resultant degree of disability. Good statistical data comparing the various surgical procedures (electrode placement on skin, along peripheral nerves, and along spinal cord pathways; destruction of pain pathways in the CNS; making lesions in the frontal lobe; ablating the pituitary gland) are difficult to find. (**Ref.** 9, pp. 104–111)

435. (E) Very few intracranial tissues are pain sensitive; thus, the cranium, brain parenchyma, most of the dura, most of the pia arachnoid, ventricular ependyma, and choroid plexus are not sensitive to pain. Most head pain arises from extracerebral structures and carries a benign prognosis. (**Ref.** 9, pp. 2129–2130)

436. (A) Meningitis headache is said to be due to the reduced pain threshold of the inflamed tissues. Other systemic conditions associated with headache include fever, hypoxia, infection, foreign protein administration, hypertension, electrolyte imbalance, and unstable disorders. (**Ref.** 5, pp. 45–47)

437. (B) CSF leakage has been said to produce traction on pain-sensitive, unsupported posterior fossa tissues. This form of intracranial hypotension develops 12 hours to several days after the lumbar puncture and is characterized by headache that occurs on assuming the upright position. It begins in the posterior cervical region. (**Ref.** 9, p. 2134)

438. (B) Some have estimated that 90% of all headaches are referrable to these two categories. The basic extracranial headache mechanisms are distention of scalp arteries, sustained muscle contraction, and inflammation in or about these structures. (**Ref.** 5, pp. 44–46)

439. (A) Cluster headaches are sometimes described as being closely related to, or a variety of, migraine; not all physicians agree. A specific thermographic pattern has been reported. The attacks last 30 minutes to 2 hours, are unilateral, and affect men more than women. (**Ref.** 5, p. 775; **Ref.** 9, p. 2131)

440. (C) Various research approaches indicate a possible relationship of serotonin metabolites to migraine. During the migraine headache, platelets undergo a release reaction that results in a reduction of serotonin content. During the attack-free interval, platelet aggregability increases. (**Ref.** 5, pp. 773–775)

441. (C) This condition is often found in association with emotional tension. There is also much overlap between the symptoms of common migraine and tension headaches; many patients suffer from both. Headaches may be constant for months. Amitryptiline is often effective. (**Ref.** 9, p. 2132)

442. (E) Nevertheless, it is felt that the headaches are due primarily to vascular and muscle contraction causes. Hypertensive headaches are characterized by early-morning, usually throbbing, occipital pain that responds to the treatment of the hypertension. (**Ref.** 9, p. 2132)

443. (B) A painful stimulus in a tooth usually causes local toothache but may cause referred pain remote from that tooth. Injection of procaine into the tissues about the suspected tooth may reduce the intensity of, or eliminate, the headache of dental origin. (**Ref.** 9, p. 2134)

444. (E) The fifth, seventh, ninth, and tenth cranial nerves contribute to the sensory innervation of the ear. Primary ear disease is relatively infrequent, but important, as a source of headache because it almost always indicates inflammation or destructive disease. (**Ref.** 9, p. 2134)

445. (A) It has been said that with a battery of such tests, sensory neural defects can be subdivided into cochlear and retrocochlear types with about 70% or more accuracy. In sensorineural hearing loss, diplacusis and recruitment are common with cochlear lesions; tone decay usually accompanies eighth nerve involvement. (**Ref.** 9, pp. 2117–2119)

446. (C) Cholesteatoma can cause mixed conductive-sensorineural loss. However, obstruction in the external auditory meatus is the most common cause of conductive hearing loss, due to impacted cerumen. (**Ref.** 9, p. 2118)

447. (D) Sudden unilateral sensorineural loss, occasionally profound, occurs with various viral diseases. Acute unilateral deafness usually has a cochlear basis. Mumps hearing loss is unilateral in 65% of the cases. (**Ref.** 9, p. 2119; **Ref.** 5, p. 109)

448. (B) It is not yet known why a young adult treated "successfully" for congenital syphilis subsequently develops these changes; treatment failure rather than autoimmune responses or a late fibrotic reaction is possible. The Hutchinson triad comprises interstitial keratitis, deformed teeth, and hearing loss; the triad is seldom complete, and congenital neurosyphilis in North America is now rare. (**Ref.** 5, p. 157; **Ref.** 9, p. 1718)

449. (C) This very common cause of deafness has been reported to respond well to surgery in more than 90% of the cases. In otosclerosis, there is overgrowth and calcification of the annual ligament, which attaches the stapes to the oval window. (**Ref. 9, pp. 2118–2119**)

450. (D) The site of the lesion is disputed; perhaps it is near the cerebral aqueduct or in the ciliary ganglion. Some add another abnormality to this syndrome, namely, a patchy atrophy and depigmentation of the iris. (**Ref. 4, pp. 46–47**)

451. (B) There may be symptoms, or the patient may complain of sudden blurred vision. The Holmes-Adie syndrome is not uncommon and is important because, though itself benign, it may be confused with Argyll-Robertson pupil or other serious pupillary abnormalities. (**Ref. 4, p. 47**)

452. (E) At the pontine level, lesions may affect the trigeminal motor root, causing ipsilateral weakness and wasting of the muscles of mastication. Where there is bilateral masticatory muscle paralysis, the jaw hangs open, as may occur in the late stages of motor neuron disease and in some cases of myasthenia gravis. (**Ref. 4, p. 61**)

453. (A) In hysterical paralysis, the tongue cannot be pushed to the "paralyzed" side. Tongue apraxia may be encountered. (**Ref. 5, p. 428**)

454. (E) Tinnitus is the earliest symptom of involvement of the eighth cranial nerve; it may precede objective hearing impairment by months or years; it is not caused by central lesions. (**Ref. 5, pp. 32–33**)

455. (D) Chvostek's sign is also sometimes found in tuberculosis and other conditions; Trousseau's sign is found only in tetany. In hypomagnesemia, tetany does not respond to correction of the accompanying hypocalcemia unless the magnesium deficit is also corrected. (**Ref. 5, p. 732**)

456. (D) In organic hemiparesis the pressure from the contralateral heel increases, but not in hysteria (Hoover's sign). Femoral nerve hysterical paralysis is also diagnosed by the presence of the knee jerk. (**Ref.** 5, p. 437)

457. **(B)**   The patient's spontaneous description of pain differentiates it from other kinds of facial pain. Eating or talking may set it off. It rarely occurs at night. This condition has been related by some to compression of the nerve by arteries or veins of the posterior fossa; occasionally it may be a symptom of a Gasserian ganglion tumor, multiple sclerosis, or a brainstem infarct. (**Ref.** 9, p. 2135; **Ref.** 5, pp. 419–420)

458. **(B)**   Although this is a much rarer condition, the pain is similar in quality to that of trigeminal neuralgia. The cardiac effects are due to the intense afferent discharge over the glossopharyngeal nerve. Carbamazepine often helps relieve the pain. (**Ref.** 9, p. 2135)

459. **(B)**   The pains are analogous to those of trigeminal and glossopharyngeal neuralgia. As in those two disorders, the pain usually responds to carbamazepine. There is no surgical therapy. (**Ref.** 9, p. 2136)

460. **(B)**   In this condition, there is a history of acute trauma, dysesthesia, and trophic changes in the involved limb. If an injury has not involved a peripheral nerve, the "reflex sympathetic dystrophy" may be called "post-traumatic painful osteoporosis." "Sudeck's atrophy," "post-traumatic spreading neuralgia," "minor causalgia," "shoulder-hand syndrome," or "reflex dystrophy." Lidocaine and sympathetic block may help. (**Ref.** 9, p. 2136)

461. **(A)**   Head tremor rarely, if ever, occurs in parkinsonism; instead, there is tremor of the lips, tongue, and jaw. (**Ref.** 5, p. 657)

462. **(A)**   It appears to be an autosomal dominant trait. It usually occurs in families. (**Ref.** 5, p. 657)

463. **(A)**   It is important to distinguish this condition from parkinsonism. Propranolol and primidone are the most effective pharmacologic therapies. The condition itself is rarely sufficiently disabling to justify brain surgery. (**Ref.** 5, p. 657)

464. (B) Benign essential tremor occasionally appears in childhood, adolescence, or advanced age. Parkinsonian tremor occurs rarely as a juvenile form. (**Ref.** 5, pp. 657–658)

465. (A, B, C) Sensations of formed body distortion (metamorphopsia) and distortion of time sense occur in the Alice in Wonderland syndrome. It has been reported in a variety of causes including viral encephalitis and epilepsy but has been said to be almost pathognomonic of migraine. Localization is controversial with some authors suggesting the anterior occipital lobe, others believing it to be the posterior temporal lobe and many saying that the posterior parietal lobe (especially the non-dominant side) is the origin. The author, Lewis Carroll (Charles Lutwidge Dodgson) himself suffered from classic migraine and may also have experienced metamorphopsia. (**Ref.** 27, pp. 649–651)

466. (A, B, C) Sensations of formed body distortion (metamorphopsia) and distortion of time sense occur in the Alice in Wonderland syndrome. It has been reported in a variety of causes including viral encephalitis and epilepsy but has been said to be almost pathognomonic of migraine. Localization is controversial with some authors suggesting the anterior occipital lobe, others believing it to be the posterior temporal lobe and many saying that the posterior parietal lobe (especially the non-dominant side) is the origin. The author, Lewis Carroll (Charles Lutwidge Dodgson) himself suffered from classic migraine and may also have experienced metamorphopsia. (**Ref.** 27, pp. 649–651)

467. (A, B, C) Sensations of formed body distortion (metamorphopsia) and distortion of time sense occur in the Alice in Wonderland syndrome. It has been reported in a variety of causes including viral encephalitis and epilepsy but has been said to be almost pathognomonic of migraine. Localization is controversial with some authors suggesting the anterior occipital lobe, others believing it to be the posterior temporal lobe and many saying that the posterior parietal lobe (especially the non-dominant side) is the origin. The author, Lewis Carroll (Charles Lutwidge Dodgson) himself suffered from classic migraine and may also have experienced metamorphopsia. (**Ref.** 27, pp. 649–651)

468. (B) This group also includes sleep jerks and anxiety. (**Ref.** 9, p. 2151)

469. (A) This group also includes systemic illnesses such as uremia, hepatic, and dialysis encephalopathy. (**Ref.** 9, p. 2151)

470. (C) This group also includes spinal myoclonus. (**Ref.** 9, p. 2151)

471. (B) This group also includes toxins (eg, methylbromide, strychnine). (**Ref.** 9, p. 2151)

472. (C) This group also includes "nocturnal myoclonus" which may be associated with "restless legs syndrome." (**Ref.** 9, p. 2151)

473. (A) This often occurs with palatal myoclonus. (**Ref.** 9, p. 2151; **Ref.** 5, p. 43)

474. (D) Often associated with right hemiparesis, worse in arm. (**Ref.** 9, p. 2086)

475. (A) May be euphoric and/or paranoid. (**Ref.** 9, p. 2086)

476. (B) This may be associated with cortical sensory loss in right arm. (**Ref.** 9, p. 2086)

477. (E) May present without or with hemiparesis, worse in arm. (**Ref.** 9, p. 2086)

478. (C) Non-fluent in transcortical motor; fluent in transcortical sensory. (**Ref.** 9, p. 2086)

479. (D) Cause may remain unknown. (**Ref.** 9, p. 2090)

480. (A) Combination of choreiform movements and dementia. (**Ref.** 9, p. 2090)

481. (C) Brain imaging tests are normal. (**Ref.** 9, p. 2091)

482. (B) Most often associated with diabetes or hypertensive vascular disease. **(Ref. 9, p. 2090)**

483. (E) Seizures are rare and, if present, another etiology should be sought. **(Ref. 9, pp. 2089–2090)**

484. (D) This includes sensory, episodic, and generic memory. **(Ref. 9, pp. 2083–2084)**

485. (A) This is spared in most amnesias. **(Ref. 9, p. 2084)**

486. (E) This, too, is spared in most amnesias. **(Ref. 9, p. 2084)**

487. (C) This also occurs following herpes simplex encephalitis. **(Ref. 9, p. 2084)**

488. (B) This designates the time compartment since the amnesia began. **(Ref. 9, p. 2084)**

489. (C) Surgical damage led to the discovery of the critical contribution to memory of the hippocampal formation and its input and output stations. **(Ref. 9, p. 2084)**

490. (E) Greatest for emotionally important events. **(Ref. 9, p. 2085)**

491. (B) Caused by attacks of severe thiamine deficiency, generally in the setting of alcoholism. **(Ref. 9, p. 2084)**

492. (A) Reported originally by Bender in 1956 with additional cases reported subsequently by Fisher; etiology presumably vascular insufficiency. **(Ref. 9, p. 2085)**

493. (D) Otherwise, may resemble episodes of transient global amnesia. **(Ref. 9, p. 2085)**

13

Case Histories

DIRECTIONS (Questions 494–598): This section consists of situations, each followed by a series of questions. Study each situation, and select the ONE best answer to each question following it.

Questions 494–498: A 49-year-old man noticed the gradual onset of a progressive weakness in his hands, followed by slight thickening of his speech and difficulty in swallowing. Although an aching sensation occurred in his upper extremities, no sensory abnormalities were found on examination. Marked fasciculations and atrophy were noted at the tongue, interossei muscles, and calves. His reflexes were hyperactive and there were bilateral Babinski signs.

494. The initial diagnosis would be
- **A.** amyotrophic lateral sclerosis
- **B.** multiple sclerosis
- **C.** polyneuritis
- **D.** syringomyelia
- **E.** none of the above

495. Charcot-Marie-Tooth disease would be likely because of the
  A. absence of clubfoot
  B. absence of objective sensory loss
  C. presence of marked fasciculations, especially of the tongue
  D. age of the patient
  E. none of the above

496. In favor of myasthenia gravis would be
  A. fasciculations
  B. a negative response to neostigmine
  C. reflex abnormalities
  D. a negative Tensilon test
  E. none of the above

497. The most likely diagnosis is an illness that is
  A. relatively uncommon
  B. fatal, usually in a few years
  C. responsive to steroids
  D. more common in females
  E. characterized by remissions

498. This illness has been found to be associated with
  A. hypothyroidism
  B. cervical rib
  C. parkinsonism
  D. Arnold-Chiari malformation
  E. platybasia

Questions 499–504: A 55-year-old man, while driving an automobile, suddenly experiences an excruciating, violent, shooting pain along the left side of his face. The pain is so severe that he is forced to stop his car. The attack lasts 15 to 20 seconds but recurs several times. That evening, while being examined by his family physician, he again has an attack. He is observed to have lacrimation, injection of the conjunctiva, and an excessive flow of saliva. The exact course of this pain is described as radiating to the forehead, the eye, and the root of the nose. During the next month, these attacks appear paroxysmally. The patient undergoes personality changes and frequently talks of suicide.

499. The most likely diagnosis is
   A. schizophrenia
   B. hysteria
   C. trigeminal neuralgia
   D. facial neuralgia
   E. glaucoma

500. Another name for this disorder is
   A. manic-depressive reaction state
   B. "quick pain"
   C. tic douloureux
   D. facial palsy
   E. none of the above

501. The most common of the neuralgias is
   A. occipital
   B. glossopharyngeal
   C. Sluder's
   D. intercostal
   E. trigeminal

502. The disorder
   A. is frequently bilateral
   B. can be differentiated from tumor or aneurysm by the presence of objective sensory loss in the latter
   C. usually produces only one attack
   D. produces pain so severe that the patient usually cannot remain in one place
   E. none of the above

503. From the following list, a disease reportedly associated with this disorder is
   A. multiple sclerosis
   B. infectious hepatitis
   C. sprue
   D. kala-azar
   E. bronchopneumonia

504. Of the three types of this disorder, the division most frequently affected is the
    A. ophthalmic
    B. maxillary, unilateral
    C. mandibular, unilateral
    D. maxillary, bilateral
    E. mandibular, bilateral

Questions 505–508: A 33-year-old man sustains an injury to the right axilla. Following emergency procedures to secure hemostatis, he is examined by a neurologist. The patient is found to have an absent triceps jerk and an inability to extend the forearm, and all extensors appear to be paralyzed.

505. The nerve injured is the
    A. axillary
    B. musculocutaneous
    C. radial
    D. suprascapular
    E. median

506. The most common of all spinal nerve lesions is affection of the
    A. axillary nerve
    B. radial nerve
    C. median nerve
    D. ulnar nerve
    E. musculocutaneous nerve

507. The lesion could be located in the
    A. axilla
    B. medial part of the arm
    C. forearm
    D. elbow
    E. none of the above

508. In this patient, you would anticipate finding anesthesia of the dorsum of
    A. the fifth finger
    B. the fourth finger
    C. the third finger

D. all fingers
E. none of the above

Questions 509–514: A 23-year-old woman is hospitalized with a diagnosis of extreme exhaustion. The patient states that she has noted progressive weakness after a minimal use of her muscles. The weakness is manifested in chewing and speaking. While under observation in the hospital, she is noted to regurgitate food through her nose. After speaking for several minutes, her voice becomes nasal and gives out. Neurologic examination also reveals diplopia and ptosis of the eyelids. Psychiatric examination reveals that the patient has numerous problems. Relatives suggest to the physician in charge of the case that "the patient appears to have a different facial appearance."

509. The most likely diagnosis is
   A. "nervous exhaustion"
   B. schizophrenia
   C. psychoneurosis
   D. myasthenia gravis
   E. amyotonia

510. Which of the following would you also expect to find?
   A. sensory disturbances
   B. fibrillation
   C. sphincter disturbances
   D. atrophies
   E. none of the above

511. Of the following drugs, which would reduce her symptoms to a persistent functional level?
   A. tranquilizers
   B. neostigmine
   C. quinine
   D. Tensilon
   E. A and C

512. The affected muscles are generally stronger in the
- **A.** morning
- **B.** afternoon
- **C.** evening
- **D.** B and C
- **E.** no correlations

513. Specific treatment should include
- **A.** shock therapy
- **B.** thyroid extract
- **C.** atropine
- **D.** Mestinon
- **E.** Tensilon

514. A drug that severely aggravates the symptoms in this illness is
- **A.** ephedrine
- **B.** quinine
- **C.** glycine
- **D.** ambenomium
- **E.** none of the above

Questions 515–521: A 42-year-old man is admitted to the hospital with a tentative diagnosis of syringomelia. The patient states that he first sought medical help when he bruised his right hand but felt no pain. Examination revealed a loss of pain and temperature sensation in both hands. He also admitted to having been treated for syphilis as a youth. The hands appeared red but not edematous; hyperhydrosis was found. No loss of position or vibratory sensations was detected. After extensive neurologic examinations, it was felt that the patient did not have tabes dorsalis.

515. The most likely diagnosis is
- **A.** tabes dorsalis
- **B.** general paresis
- **C.** syringomyelia
- **D.** hysteria
- **E.** brain abscess

516. The prognosis for this patient is
- **A.** excellent
- **B.** good

    C. unfavorable

    D. impossible to predict

    E. a pattern of remission and exacerbation

517. The etiology is due

    A. most often to bacteria

    B. occasionally to spirochetes

    C. to viruses

    D. to vascular accidents

    E. to an unknown cause

518. To differentiate this from amyotrophic lateral sclerosis, appropriate tests should include

    A. electroencephalograms

    B. pneumoencephalograms

    C. vertebral angiograms

    D. amytal tests

    E. none of the above

519. If this patient developed fasciculations of the tongue and paralysis of the vocal cords, the disease has extended to the

    A. cervical spinal cord

    B. medulla oblongata

    C. pons

    D. globus pallidus

    E. hypothalamus

520. If this disorder is syringomyelia, one would expect to find which of the following changes in the wrist, biceps, and triceps reflexes?

    A. lost

    B. hypoactive

    C. hyperactive

    D. clonic

    E. normal

521. The treatment should include
  A. thyroid
  B. vitamin B_{12}
  C. vitamin B_{12}
  D. adrenalin
  E. none of the above

Questions 522–524: A 49-year-old woman presents with dysesthesias of the hands and feet. Examination reveals absent deep tendon reflexes and loss of vibratory and positional sensation. The disease progresses to a spastic ataxic paraplegia. Several months after the onset of her illness, Babinski signs develop bilaterally. Within six months the patient dies because of cachexia and advanced cord disintegration. During the entire course of this patient's illness, no pupillary disturbance or ocular palsies were observed. Repeated blood and CSF Wasserman tests were negative.

522. The most likely diagnosis is
  A. Friedreich's ataxia
  B. tabes dorsalis
  C. multiple sclerosis
  D. subacute combined "degeneration" or sclerosis
  E. general paresis

523. The most significant diagnostic procedure would have been
  A. electroencephalograms performed serially while the patient was asleep
  B. electromyography after exercise
  C. CT or MRI
  D. skin and muscle biopsies of the legs, arms, and trunk
  E. hematologic surveys

524. The pathologic process in the spinal cord seems to be primarily involving the
  A. posterior and lateral columns
  B. spinocerebellar tracts
  C. anterior horn cells
  D. column of Clarke
  E. ependyma

Questions 525–530: An 18-year-old male student presents with a history of several "attacks," lasting for 18 hours, or gradual ascending and rapidly progressive flaccid paralysis. The patient states that the lower extremities are involved first and later the upper extremities. The boy is afebrile during these attacks. A lumbar puncture is performed, but no abnormalities of the spinal fluid are found. The patient is hospitalized, and during one of these attacks he is found to have absent deep tendon reflexes and a loss of electrical responses. The patient's mother states that "the boy's uncle died of brain trouble." However, records to uncover the etiology of the uncle's disease are unobtainable.

525. The most likely diagnosis is
  A. Landry's paralysis
  B. hysterical neurosis
  C. acute poliomyelitis
  D. familial periodic paralysis
  E. tick paralysis

526. Which of the following is not compatible with the diagnosis?
  A. age of the patient
  B. spinal fluid findings
  C. lack of fever
  D. absent deep tendon reflexes
  E. all facts given are compatible

527. During an attack, one would most likely find
  A. low serum potassium
  B. high serum potassium
  C. low blood sugar
  D. high blood sugar
  E. none of the above

528. During an attack the patient may benefit from
  A. adrenalin IV
  B. adrenalin IM
  C. 5% dextrose water IV
  D. 10% dextrose water IV
  E. none of the above

529. At the height of an attack the patient would most likely resemble a patient with a sudden attack of
    A. brain abscess
    B. acute poliomyelitis
    C. psychomotor epilepsy
    D. vitamin E deficiency
    E. Sydenham's chorea

530. Attacks may be prevented with
    A. potassium chloride
    B. parathyroid extract
    C. adrenalin
    D. testosterone
    E. none of the above

Questions 531–535: A 27-year-old man is admitted to the hospital with paralysis of the right arm. The patient states that he had been in excellent health, except for a mild cold two weeks prior to the onset of his present illness. He thought that there may have been a change in his bowel habits. Examination reveals a flaccid paralysis of the right arm, with pain on passive motion, hyperesthesia, and hypoactivity of the biceps tendon reflex. The examiner gets the impression that there is some rigidity of the neck, but meningeal signs are not elicited. No other abnormal neurologic findings are obtained. A lumbar puncture reveals clear spinal fluid under moderate pressure. The laboratory analysis of this fluid: 20 polymorphonuclear leukocytes, normal sugar, and increased protein. The white cell count of the blood is 12,000/mL.

531. The most likely diagnosis is
    A. tuberculous meningitis
    B. acute anterior poliomyelitis
    C. multiple neuritis
    D. tick paralysis
    E. right cerebral brain abscess

532. Least compatible with the diagnosis is
    A. a history of mild cold
    B. type of paralysis
    C. rigidity of the neck
    D. normal spinal fluid sugar
    E. sphincter dysfunction

533. Which of the following determinations would be most useful in the diagnosis?
   A. neutralizing antibodies of the spinal fluid
   B. blood cultures
   C. x-rays of the vertebral columns
   D. ASLO titers
   E. none of the above would help much

534. From the neurological observations, the lesion is most likely located in the
   A. spinal cord
   B. medulla oblongata
   C. pons
   D. cerebellum
   E. cerebrum

535. Treatment of the patient should include
   A. isolation for four weeks
   B. strict bed rest
   C. Salk vaccine or Sabin vaccine
   D. gamma globulin
   E. A and B

Questions 536–538: A 28-year-old bartender is admitted to the hospital with symmetric gangrene of the distal phalanges. The history reveals that the patient's disorder began with dysesthesias of the fingers, which looked pale and felt cold. The patient experienced intense pain at that time. About 20 minutes after this attack, the phalanges became cyanotic and the pain became more intense. The cyanosis was followed by gangrene. The same sequence of events took place a second time before the patient sought medical attention. A urinalysis revealed intermittent albuminuria and paroxysmal hemoglobinuria.

536. The most likely diagnosis is
   A. Buerger's disease
   B. erythromelalgia
   C. acroparesthesia
   D. Raynaud's disease
   E. leprosy

537. Pathologic specimens of the digits will show
  A. normal veins
  B. normal arteries
  C. sclerosis of veins
  D. sclerosis of arteries
  E. A and B

538. The prognosis for life is
  A. good
  B. fair
  C. poor
  D. grave
  E. completely unpredictable

Questions 539–543: A 32-year-old man was bitten by a wild fox. He was taken to the emergency room of a nearby hospital, where the wound is debrided. He was given 2000 units of T.A.T. and 1.2 million units of penicillin. Inasmuch as there has not been a reported case of rabies in the area for over 10 years, antirabies therapy was not started. The patient did well and returned to work. One month later the patient became quite irritable and developed malaise, anorexia, and headache. Mild spasms of the larynx and pharynx developed, and he had precordial pain. The patient was hospitalized and clinically progressed to the various stages of paralytic rabies. He died five days after admission to the hospital.

539. The disease is caused by
  A. bacteria
  B. spirochete
  C. virus
  D. rickettsia
  E. fungus

540. Other clinical features of rabies do not include
  A. delirium and hallucinations
  B. paresthesias near the bite
  C. intense thirst
  D. bradycardia
  E. none of the above

541. The mortality for untreated persons is about
- **A.** 10%
- **B.** 30%
- **C.** 50%
- **D.** 70%
- **E.** over 70%

542. Characteristic lesions are found in the
- **A.** medulla oblongata but not Ammon's horn
- **B.** pons but not the spinal ganglia
- **C.** cord and cortex but not the spinal ganglia
- **D.** Ammon's horn but not the spinal ganglia
- **E.** none of the above

543. Paralytic types of rabies are more apt to follow bites on the
- **A.** leg
- **B.** neck
- **C.** head
- **D.** ear
- **E.** lip

Questions 544–550: A 62-year-old man is admitted to the hospital for diagnostic evaluation of loss of libido. Three months prior to admission, he developed severe leg pains and was advised that he had "sciatica." Two months later he had several episodes of retching, vomiting, and abdominal pains. The patient lost 14 pounds at that time. These problems suddenly subsided, his appetite returned, and he regained 10 pounds. Examination on admission to the hospital revealed impairment of position and vibratory sensation, primarily of the toes. A positive Romberg sign was present. The patient appeared ataxic when his eyes were closed. Knee jerks and ankle jerks were markedly diminished. Pupil examination showed anisocoria, constriction on convergence, and no reaction to light.

544. The most likely diagnosis is
- **A.** general paresis
- **B.** tabes
- **C.** multiple sclerosis
- **D.** multiple neuritis
- **E.** combined sclerosis

545. Differentiation among all the choices in question **544** can be made by which of the following tests?
   A. gastric analysis
   B. GI series
   C. urine electrophoresis
   D. lumbar puncture
   E. none of the above

546. The history of pain with this disease is
   A. very unusual
   B. occasionally found
   C. almost always present
   D. never observed
   E. found in 30% to 40% of the cases

547. The gastric crises described result from an inflammatory process involving sympathetic rami of the
   A. lower sacral roots
   B. lower dorsal roots
   C. vagal roots
   D. upper cervical roots
   E. none of the above

548. The impairment of position and vibratory sensation is due to degeneration of
   A. anterior horn cells
   B. intermediate cell columns
   C. posterior columns of Goll and Burdach
   D. dorsal root ganglia
   E. none of the above

549. The reactions of the pupil as described occur
   A. only in this disease
   B. only with brain tumors
   C. only in multiple sclerosis
   D. in several disorders
   E. none of the above

550. The ataxia is due to lesions in the
   A. spinal cord
   B. medulla oblongata

C. pons
D. cerebellum
E. cerebral cortex

Questions 551–555: A 64-year-old candy store owner notices a tremor in the fingers of his right hand. The tremor is fine and rhythmic and appears to stop on voluntary movements. The patient's private physician also detects a tremor of the jaw and tongue. However, no paralyses can be found on thorough examination. Gradually, the patient develops a posture in which the right arm does not swing when walking. The patient has a sleepy expression, and the face becomes rigid or mask-like. Several months later the patient walks as if all his muscles were rigid, and with great hesitation.

551. The most likely diagnosis is
    A. paralysis agitans
    B. general paresis
    C. tabes
    D. hysteria
    E. Wilson's disease

552. The disease is limited to persons
    A. over 60 years
    B. over 40 years
    C. over 20 years
    D. no age limit
    E. over 70 years

553. In taking a history from this patient, inquiries should be made about ingestion of
    A. chlorpromazine
    B. thyroid extract
    C. heroin
    D. aspirin
    E. lead paint

554. Pathologic examination in the above case would most likely show
  A. hemorrhage into the basal ganglia
  B. lues of the substantia nigra
  C. neoplastic invasion of the globus pallidus
  D. no direct etiologic factor
  E. hemorrhage into the striatum

555. Curative therapy consists of
  A. antihistamines and psychotherapy
  B. hyoscine hydrobromide and belladonna
  C. neither A nor B
  D. codeine and pagitane hydrochloride
  E. Parsidol and vitamin B_6

Questions 556–559: A patient sustains an injury which produces hemisection of his spinal cord. For the following questions, the level of injury is not an important factor.

556. This lesion is seen most completely in
  A. malignant tumors
  B. benign tumors
  C. aneurysm of anterior spinal arteries
  D. knife wounds
  E. viral infections

557. Deep reflexes and muscle tone are
  A. increased on the same side
  B. decreased on the same side
  C. increased on the opposite side
  D. decreased on the opposite side
  E. no change in deep reflexes

558. Ipsilateral impairment of point discrimination results from
  A. injury to anterior columns
  B. injury to posterior columns
  C. injury to medial columns
  D. injury to lateral columns
  E. it does not occur with cord lesions

559. Such a lesion is called the
  A. syringomyelia syndrome
  B. Brown-Sequard syndrome
  C. paraplegic syndrome
  D. low back syndrome
  E. none of the above

Questions 560–565: Identify the following spinal cord lesions by the pathological description.

  A. Multiple sclerosis
  B. Amyotrophic lateral sclerosis
  C. Combined sclerosis (subacute combined degeneration)
  D. Anterior poliomyelitis
  E. Syringomyelia
  F. Hydromyelia
  G. Brown-Sequard syndrome
  H. Spina bifida

560. Tubular cavitation of the spinal cord usually beginning within the cervical canal and generally extending ultimately over many segments.

561. Enormously dilated remnant of the fetal central canal.

562. Large motor neurons of the anterior horn cells are reduced in number; anterior root size is decreased. Corticospinal tracts are degenerated.

563. Demyelinated areas vary in size from small lesions of the posterior or lateral funiculi to almost complete loss of myelin in an entire cross section of the cord.

564. White matter is much more affected than gray matter. Demyelination is symmetric; to a lesser extent, axonal loss is found, especially in the posterior and lateral columns. Lesions appear first in the thoracic posterior columns.

565. Large motor cells are especially involved; the degeneration is accompanied by an inflammatory meningeal reaction. To a lesser extent, changes may be found also in the posterior horn, posterior root ganglion, and elsewhere in the central nervous system.

Questions 566–569: On examination, a patient has difficulty seeing finger motion or a red match at the right side of his right eye and the left side of his left eye.

566. The lesion is located in the
    A. retina
    B. optic nerve
    C. optic chiasm
    D. geniculate body
    E. none of the above

567. The defect is called
    A. bitemporal hemianopsia
    B. left homonymous hemianopsia
    C. binasal hemianopsia
    D. complete homonymous hemianopsia
    E. total blindness

568. The defect is most often produced by
    A. bullet wounds
    B. tumors
    C. vascular accidents
    D. infections
    E. degenerative metabolic diseases

569. Associated abnormalities caused by this group of lesions include
    A. changes in skin but not hair
    B. depressed function of the adrenals but not of the thyroid
    C. changes in the viscera and subcutaneous tissues, but not in sexual activity
    D. "tufting" and kyphosis
    E. none of the above

Questions 570–573: A patient is asked to close her eyes. The left eye can be closed only partly and the left side of her mouth droops slightly; a small amount of saliva is noted at the left side of her mouth. She is not able to taste salt on the left side of her tongue.

570. The disorder is known as
   A. Horner's syndrome
   B. trigeminal neuralgia
   C. Bell's palsy
   D. facial neuralgia
   E. rabies

571. The characteristic facial appearance results from injury of the
   A. maxillary division of the trigeminal nerve
   B. ophthalmic division of the trigeminal nerve
   C. vagus nerve
   D. facial nerve
   E. A and B

572. Concerning closure of the eyes, the patient cannot close the eye on the
   A. opposite side reflexly or voluntarily
   B. side of the lesion voluntarily but can reflexly
   C. opposite side reflexly but can voluntarily
   D. side of the lesion reflexly but can voluntarily
   E. none of these statements are true in their entirety

573. The prognosis for return of function is
   A. very grave
   B. poor
   C. fair
   D. good
   E. no single case has been reported for return of function

Questions 574–577: The patient presents with a chief complaint of "double vision." When he tries to look to his right, the examiner notes that the left eye adducts and the right eye is in the midline or slightly adducted. When the patient looks straight ahead at the examiner, the right eye adducts slightly and the left eye is in the midline.

574. The eye muscle paralyzed is the
   A. right external rectus
   B. left external rectus
   C. right internal rectus
   D. left internal rectus
   E. none of the above

575. The diplopia will be most marked when the patient attempts to look
   A. to his left
   B. to his right
   C. downward
   D. upward
   E. direction has no effect

576. At rest, the patient has
   A. external squint
   B. photophobia
   C. strabismus
   D. myopia
   E. no abnormality

577. The patient sees double because of
   A. delay in transmission time from the affected eye
   B. conscious willing of double sight to compensate for physical disability
   C. "image blocking" by the retina of the affected eye
   D. "image blocking" at the optic chiasm
   E. none of the above

Questions 578–581: The patient, age one month, presents with vomiting and irritability. The examiner finds that the skull is enlarged and the fontanels are widened. The face is normal in size but appears small relative to the enlarged head. The orbits are displaced downward resulting in exophthalmos and scleral prominence.

578. The most likely diagnosis is
- **A.** oxycephaly
- **B.** scaphocephaly
- **C.** hydrocephalus
- **D.** encephalocele
- **E.** mental retardation

579. The most enlightening procedure would be
- **A.** air encephalography or CT
- **B.** electroencephalography
- **C.** hematocrit
- **D.** skull x-rays
- **E.** lumbar puncture

580. The patient should be managed or treated with
- **A.** x-radiation
- **B.** iodine
- **C.** anticoagulants
- **D.** subdural aspiration
- **E.** none of the above

581. This disorder may be caused by
- **A.** *Hemophilus influenzae* but not venous sinus thrombosis
- **B.** staphylococcus but not brain tumor
- **C.** tuberculosis but not congenital absence of the aqueduct of Sylvius
- **D.** congenital absence of the foramina of exit but not of the aqueduct of Sylvius
- **E.** none of the above

Questions 582–585: Following injury, examination of a patient in the anatomical position discloses cutaneous loss in the right upper extremity involving the right fifth finger, part of the right fourth finger, the inner aspect of the right hand (dorsal and volar), and the inner aspect of the right forearm.

582. The lesion is located in the
   A. brachial plexus
   B. medulla oblongata
   C. pons
   D. ulnar nerve
   E. lumbar plexus

583. This might well be accompanied by
   A. mydriasis
   B. miosis
   C. exophthalmos
   D. widened palpebral fissure
   E. none of the above

584. The cervical nerve root involved is
   A. C1
   B. C2
   C. C3
   D. C4
   E. none of the above

585. The area of skin supplied by fibers of any one posterior root is called a
   A. neurotome
   B. cryotome
   C. myotome
   D. dermatome
   E. biotome

Questions 586–587: An infant is found to have an occipital skull defect with a sac-like protrusion of the overlying skin. Studies show cerebral tissue is present in the protrusion.

586. The most likely diagnosis is
   A. craniotabes
   B. hydrocephalus
   C. encephalocele
   D. myelocele
   E. craniosynostosis

587. The defect is usually
   A. midline
   B. over the parietal bone
   C. over the frontal bone
   D. over the temporal bone
   E. not a bony defect

Questions 588–590: When asked to smile, a patient appeared to be snarling. His voice was weak and nasal. These signs would be most pronounced in the evening and would temporarily improve after a night's rest.

588. His appearance is characteristic of
   A. congenital lues
   B. myasthenia gravis
   C. bilateral middle cerebral artery aneurysms
   D. psychoneurosis
   E. multiple sclerosis

589. In this illness, one often encounters
   A. unilateral sensory deficit
   B. bilateral sensory deficit
   C. no sensory deficit
   D. hyperactive deep tendon reflexes
   E. unilateral or bilateral Babinski's reflex

590. Most often there are
  A. fibrillations
  B. atrophy
  C. sphincter disturbances
  D. hyperpathia
  E. none of the above

Questions 591-594: A patient complained of severe back pain at the left lower thoracic region. Examination revealed a cluster of vesicles in approximately the same region; later on, a scab was noted which, after desquamation, left a pigmented scar.

591. The lesion is caused by a
  A. spirochete
  B. virus
  C. bacterium
  D. rickettsia
  E. none of the above

592. It may be found in association with
  A. tumor but not uremia
  B. meningitis but not leukemia
  C. uremia but not arsenic intoxication
  D. tuberculosis
  E. none of the above

593. Residua of the illness
  A. are almost invariably easy to manage
  B. are often very difficult to manage
  C. usually respond well to antibiotics
  D. should be treated early by avulsion of nerves
  E. can usually be prevented by the use of gamma globulin

594. This illness
  A. does not affect the peripheral nerves
  B. affects the spinal cord, especially the anterior horn
  C. affects the roots, especially the anterior
  D. affects the dorsal root ganglia and the sensory ganglia of cranial nerves
  E. none of the above

Questions 595–598: The patient presents with a chief complaint of "double vision." When he tries to look to his left, the examiner notes that the right eye is in the midline, whereas the left eye is in abduction. The right eyelid is drooping and the right pupil is larger than the left pupil. When he looks upward, the right eye is in the midline, whereas the left eye is in the up position. The right eyelid is still lower than the left and the right pupil is larger than the left pupil.

595. The cranial nerve involvement includes the right
   A. third nerve
   B. fourth nerve
   C. sixth nerve
   D. third and sixth nerves
   E. fourth and sixth nerves

596. Lesions in this area are most frequently encountered in
   A. slow-growing neoplasms
   B. vascular disease
   C. platybasia
   D. psychoneurosis
   E. uremia

597. Of the following, if a single lesion is present, one would most likely find
   A. weakness of the right upper extremity
   B. weakness of both left extremities
   C. right homonymous hemianopsia
   D. impaired vibration sense in the left lower extremity
   E. impaired vibration sense in the right lower extremity

598. Particularly important in diagnosis would be
   A. myelography
   B. visual field testing
   C. creatine levels
   D. angiography
   E. none of the above

Answers and Discussion

494. (A) The multiple motor defects, with signs of anterior horn cell disease and no sensory or trophic abnormalities, would tend to exclude the others. (**Ref.** 5, pp. 682–686)

495. (E) Charcot-Marie-Tooth disease is much more common in the first and second decades of life. Charcot-Marie-Tooth disease usually includes impairment of sensation in a "stocking-and-glove" distribution. (**Ref.** 5, pp. 604–605)

496. (E) Ocular involvement is the most common presenting symptom in myasthenia gravis. For all practical purposes, a positive response to Tensilon (edrophonium) or neostigmine is diagnostic of myasthenia gravis. (**Ref.** 5, pp. 702–703)

497. (B) Extremes of duration in one study ranged from a few months to 10 years. Most often, death occurs within five years of onset, especially when there are both upper and lower motor neuron signs. (**Ref.** 5, p. 685)

498. (C) There is a very high incidence of amyotrophic lateral sclerosis (ALS) among the Chamorro Indians on Guam (50 to 100 times greater than anywhere else in the world). On Guam (not in the United States), ALS is often associated with components of the Parkinson-dementia complex. (**Ref.** 5, p. 683)

499. (C) Glaucoma may appear suddenly, but the pain is usually limited to the eyeball and orbit, the globe is tense, and the pupil is dilated and fixed to light. The pain of herpes zoster may simulate that of trigeminal neuralgia, but the appearance of the vesicles establishes the correct diagnosis. (**Ref. 5, pp.** 419–421)

500. (C) The pain may be so severe that mental changes occur; there may be depression and even suicide. Morphine addiction is rare. Most often, the second and third divisions of the nerve are involved. (**Ref.** 5, pp. 419–421)

501. (E) In glossopharyngeal neuralgia, swallowing rather than chewing starts an attack. In addition, in glossopharyngeal neuralgia, spraying the tonsillar region with local anesthetic helps establish the diagnosis. (**Ref.** 5, p. 421)

502. (B) In tumor or aneurysm, one looks for loss of sensation in the trigeminal region, especially corneal anesthesia and weakness of the muscles of mastication. Also, other cranial nerves may be involved. Trigeminal neuralgia is usually unilateral. The patient avoids movement or touching the area and lives in fear of the next attack. (**Ref.** 5, p. 420)

503. (A) In most instances, no cause can be found. Pain typical of trigeminal neuralgia has occasionally occurred in patients with brain stem lesions due to multiple sclerosis. (**Ref.** 5, p. 419)

504. (B) The affection is nearly always unilateral; the ophthalmic division is involved least often. Pain originally confined to one division may spread to one or both of the other divisions. (**Ref.** 5, p. 420)

505. (C) In the differential diagnosis, lead palsy is usually bilateral and often spares the brachioradialis; hysteria usually shows no atrophy or electric changes. Involvement of the brachioradialis produces weakness of forearm flexion. (**Ref.** 5, p. 429)

506. (B) A variety of traumata, with or without fracture or dislocation, may injure this nerve. Cuts, gunshot wounds, pressure from crutches, or other pressure (eg, "Saturday night palsy") can injure it. (**Ref.** 5, p. 429)

507. (A) Involvement of all extensors, including the triceps, places the lesion in the axilla. Radial nerve lesions in the axilla are usually accompanied by evidence of injury to other nerves in the region. (**Ref.** 5, p. 429)

508. (E) Because the sensory nerves overlap, impaired sensation is usually limited to the dorsum of the thumb and index finger and the first interosseous space. Causalgia rarely follows partial injury to the nerve. (**Ref.** 5, p. 429)

509. (D) The Tensilon (edrophonium) test (or the neostigmine test) is generally positive in myasthenia gravis, except for occasional cases of myasthenia confined to the ocular muscles. The differential diagnosis includes all diseases that are accompanied by weakness of oropharyngeal or limb muscles. (**Ref.** 5, pp. 701–702)

510. (E) There is also no reaction of degeneration. Reflexes are preserved even in muscles that are weak. (**Ref.** 5, p. 700)

511. (B) Tensilon is used diagnostically only; neostigmine is used diagnostically and therapeutically. Certain antibiotics, such as neomycin, impair acetylcholine release. (**Ref.** 5, pp. 702–703)

512. (A) At least early in the course, weak muscles do regain their power after a period of rest. The weakness also varies from day to day or over longer periods. (**Ref.** 5, pp. 699–700)

513. (D) Ambenonium (Mytelase), steroids, and, in some cases, thymectomy are also used. In about 10% of myasthenia patients, myasthenic crisis occurs; this is the need for assisted ventilation. (**Ref.** 5, pp. 702–703)

514. (B) This, therefore, was formerly used as a diagnostic test. Any respiratory depressant drug should be avoided in myasthenia. (**Ref.** 4, p. 443)

515. (C) The disease typically involves segmental sensory loss (mainly or only) of pain and temperature, plus segmental atrophy. Neurogenic arthropathies (Charcot joints) may affect the shoulder, elbow, or wrist. (**Ref.** 5, pp. 687–688)

516. (C) However, the disease sometimes apparently becomes arrested; if bulbar symptoms occur, a more rapid course is expected. Radiotherapy to halt extension of the syringomyelic cavity is of doubtful benefit. **(Ref. 5, p. 690)**

517. (E) It is felt to be most likely congenital developmental; it is frequently associated with other congenital defects. Familial cases have been described. **(Ref. 5, pp. 688–689)**

518. (E) Amyotrophic lateral sclerosis shows increased deep reflexes and no sensory loss. Myelography or metrizamide-CT myelography shows cord abnormalities. **(Ref. 5, p. 690)**

519. (B) The disease may also extend further to the pons and peduncles, and reportedly even to the basal ganglia. Syringobulbia also causes dysphagia, pharyngeal, and palatal weakness, along with nystagmus. **(Ref. 5, p. 688)**

520. (A) In later stages, involvement of the pyramidal tracts may cause hyperactive deep tendon reflexes in the lower extremities and a Babinski sign. Intermediolateral cell column damage to the sympathetic neurons may cause Horner's syndrome. **(Ref. 5, pp. 687–688)**

521. (E) There is no satisfactory treatment. Surgery might possibly be of benefit in those cases with associated abnormalities of the foramen magnum, for example. Radiotherapy might be helpful when an intramedullary tumor is associated with the syrinx. **(Ref. 5, p. 690)**

522. (D) Optic atrophy with visual field dysfunction may be found early; mental changes are also described. The disease usually starts in the dorsal column of the thoracic cord; therefore, the first symptoms typically include paresthesias of the feet. **(Ref. 5, pp. 691–694)**

523. (E) Diagnosis can be established by the failure of absorption of orally administered radioactive vitamin B_{12} (Schilling test); recent investigations concern the presence of serum antibodies to gastric parietal cells. Nonspecific abnormalities may help in diagnosis, namely, elevated serum lactic dehydrogenase or elevated unconjugated serum bilirubin. (**Ref.** 5, p. 693)

524. **(A)**   The involvement may be diffuse and may also affect the spinocerebellar tracts, anterior horn cells, column of Clarke, posterior roots, and peripheral nerves. The white matter is more involved than the gray. (**Ref.** 5, p. 692)

525. **(D)**   This disorder may now be subdivided into three types, depending upon the level of serum potassium. Others say that at least two types can be distinguished and that there are probably more. (**Ref.** 5, pp. 720–723)

526. **(E)**   The age here is more compatible with the low-potassium type than with the high-potassium type. Yet, the low-potassium type has been reported as early as the age of four and as late as the sixth decade. (**Ref.** 5, pp. 720–723)

527. **(A)**   The low-potassium type is the most common; the normal-potassium type is the least common. Potassium values may be 3.0 mEq/L or lower. (**Ref.** 5, pp. 721–722)

528. **(E)**   Food, especially carbohydrates, worsens the low-potassium attack but relieves the high-potassium attack. Cold may induce an attack in either the low-potassium or the high-potassium type. (**Ref.** 5, p. 721)

529. **(B)**   The diagnosis is based upon familial occurrence of transient attacks of weakness. In sporadic cases, other causes of hypokalemia, the differential diagnosis includes uremia, Addison's disease, spironolactone excess, and excessive intake of potassium. (**Ref.** 5, p. 722)

530. **(A)**   Oral acetazolamide seems to be the most effective therapy currently available. Treatment with acetazolamide may also improve the fixed weakness between attacks. (**Ref.** 5, pp. 722–723)

531. **(B)**   In sporadic cases, the prodromal period cannot be properly evaluated, so the diagnosis is made only after the onset of paralysis. Paralysis, when it occurs, usually but not always develops be-

tween the second and fifth day after the onset of signs and involvement of the nervous system. (**Ref.** 5, pp. 101–102; **Ref.** 9, pp. 2198–2200)

532. **(E)** Sphincter dysfunction has been reported but is uncommon; transient urinary bladder paralysis has been reported by some. Acute cerebellar ataxia has been observed in children. (**Ref.** 5, p. 101)

533. **(E)** The virus may be recovered from stool, throat washings, CSF, or blood. However, it is rarely recovered from the CSF. (**Ref.** 5, p. 101)

534. **(A)** Less often, there is involvement of cranial nerve motor nuclei, meninges, and even cortex. The virus has a predilection for the large motor cells, causing chromatolysis with acidophilic inclusions and necrosis of the cells. (**Ref.** 5, p. 99)

535. **(E)** Heat for muscle pain, use of a respirator in bulbar cases, rehabilitative measures. Muscle paralysis that results in stretching or malposition may require the application of removable splints. (**Ref.** 5, p. 102)

536. **(D)** With regard to Buerger's disease, it is noted that Raynaud's phenomenon may occur in it; however, Raynaud's phenomenon is rare in men. Most commonly, only the hands are affected, but the feet, nose, cheek, ears, and chin can also be involved. (**Ref.** 9, pp. 375–377)

537. **(E)** Pulsation can be felt in the larger vessels despite the changes in capillary circulation. In long-standing cases, the intima becomes thickened and the media may be hypertrophied. (**Ref.** 9, p. 376)

538. **(A)** Mild cases improve slowly or remain stationary for years. The morbidity is low and is generally limited to loss of portions of digits as a result of ulcerations. (**Ref.** 9, p. 376)

539. **(C)** The rod-shaped virus contains single-stranded RNA. The virus appears capable of infecting every warm-blooded animal. (**Ref.** 5, p. 110)

540. (D) A premonitory stage may be followed by a stage of excitement and then a stage of paralysis. The period of lethargy passes rapidly into a state of excitability in which all external stimuli are apt to cause localized twitchings or generalized convulsions. (**Ref.** 5, p. 111)

541. (E) Once the symptoms have developed, there is no specific antiviral therapy of proven value. The disease is almost fatal; a few cases with recovery have been reported. (**Ref.** 5, p. 112)

542. (E) Generalized encephalitis and myelitis are found. There is perivascular infiltration of the entire CNS with lymphocytes. (**Ref.** 5, p. 110)

543. (A) The maniacal reaction is more likely to occur with head wounds. The incidence of the disease is also highest when the wounds are severe and near the head. (**Ref.** 5, p. 111)

544. (B) One considers the combination of A-R pupils, root pains, gastric crises, posterior column involvement, impairment of knee and ankle jerks, and impotence. Other findings may include impaired superficial and deep sensation, weakness, wasting, and hypotonia of muscles. (**Ref.** 5, p. 156)

545. (E) The CSF Wassermann test can be positive in both tabes and general paresis; in each condition, there may be a pleocytosis and an increase in protein; in addition, both illnesses (taboparesis) may be present. MHT-TP and FTA-ABS tests are more specific and sensitive. (**Ref.** 4, p. 486)

546. (C) The basic pathologic process is a mild inflammation of the posterior spinal ganglia, the roots between the ganglia, and the spinal cord and the meninges. Tabes may arrest spontaneously or via treatment, but the lancinating pains and ataxia may continue. (**Ref.** 5, p. 156)

547. (B) Some distinguish between sympathetic crises with severe pain but little vomiting plus hypochlorhydria, and vagal crises with little pain but severe vomiting and hyperchlorhydria. Inappropriate operations may be performed on tabetics because of these pains; on the other hand, a tabetic may have a true surgical emergency. (**Ref.** 9, p. 2189)

548. **(C)** Other parts of the cord are not generally involved. The dorsal aspect of the cord appears wasted. Secondary demyelination of dorsal columns is found. (**Ref.** 9, p. 2188)

549. **(D)** One may also see a dilated, fixed pupil that reacts neither to light nor on convergence late in tabes with optic atrophy. One author reports that A-R pupils have been found in approximately one-half of the patients with tabes. (**Ref.** 4, p. 47; **Ref.** 5, p. 156)

550. **(A)** Early impairment of position and vibratory sensation is practically always found in tabes. This results in stumbling and progressive sensory ataxia, especially in the dark when visual compensation is imperfect. (**Ref.** 9, p. 2189)

551. **(A)** A similar picture may occur in Wilson's disease; familial incidence, corneal pigmentation, and liver cirrhosis are sought in that condition. The classic triad of symptoms in paralysis agitans is tremor, rigidity, and akinesia. (**Ref.** 5, p. 659)

552. **(D)** This may occur early in life and has been designated "juvenile paralysis agitans." It occurs in both sexes and in all races throughout the world. (**Ref.** 5, p. 658)

553. **(A)** The parkinson-like syndrome disappears with drug withdrawal, but dystonic or choreic movements may be more of a problem. Symptoms of drug-induced parkinsonism include the parkinsonian triad; dystonic movements (especially in children) involving the tongue and face; and akathisia (especially in adults)—a restless, fidgety state. (**Ref.** 5, p. 664)

554. **(D)** There are diffuse, widespread lesions in the basal ganglia and cortex; it is not always possible to distinguish the various types of parkinsonism either clinically or pathologically. Characteristically, neuronal loss and depigmentation are found in the substantia nigra, especially the zona compacta. (**Ref.** 5, p. 658)

555. **(C)** The most effective treatment currently appears to involve the administration of levodopa, especially with the concomitant

usage of one of the central anticholinergic drugs and alpha-methyllevodopa hydrazine. The goal of treatment is to promote the production of dopamine by the striatum by administering the immediate precursor, levodopa, or by direct stimulation of dopamine receptor mechanisms by ergoline derivatives. (**Ref.** 5, pp. 665–668)

556. (**D**) Clinically, especially in cord tumors, the dissociation is not nearly so clear-cut or permanent. Usually the neurologic signs are found with the upper level one or two segments below the lesion. (**Ref.** 5, p. 395)

557. (**A**) Ipsilateral weakness and other pyramidal tract signs are found. There may be ipsilateral segmental loss of sensation or weakness appropriate to the level of the lesion. (**Ref.** 5, p. 395)

558. (**B**) This is associated with ipsilateral loss of proprioceptive and vibratory sensations. There may be little loss of tactile sensation. (**Ref.** 5, p. 395)

559. (**B**) This has also been found in cases of herpes zoster and in postvaccinal and postinfectious encephalomyelitis. In herpes zoster, one may also find signs of a transverse myelitis or an ascending myelitis. (**Ref.** 5, p. 117)

560. (**E**) The cavity may be irregular; it may extend laterally and involve the pyramidal tracts. Occasionally, cavitation of the spinal cord is secondary to the presence of a tumor. (**Ref.** 4, p. 374)

561. (**F**) The tube (elongated cavity) is lined with ependymal cells of the central canal. Hydromyelia can be considered to be simple cystic expansion of the central canal of the cord. (**Ref.** 5, p. 688)

562. (**B**) Motor nuclei of the bulb are also involved. Most severely involved are the hypoglossal nucleus, the nucleus ambiguus, and the trigeminal motor nucleus. (**Ref.** 4, pp. 518–519)

563. (**A**) Practically every part of the CNS may be involved, but the gray matter is usually spared. There is widespread occurrence of patches of demyelination followed by gliosis in the white matter. (**Ref.** 4, p. 506)

564. (C) When it is diffuse, other parts of the cord may be involved, and even the posterior roots and peripheral nerves. Lesions are characterized by demyelination and the disappearance of both myelin sheaths and access cylinders, leaving vacuolated spaces separated by a fine glial meshwork. (**Ref.** 4, pp. 496–497)

565. (D) This involves anterior horn cells, occasionally cranial nerve motor nuclei, and meninges. Besides anterior horn cell degeneration, there is an inflammatory reaction with small hemorrhages in the gray matter. This consists of perivascular cuffing, mainly with lymphocytes, but with a smaller number of polymorphonuclear cells, along with diffuse gray matter infiltration by similar cells and cells of neuroglial origin. (**Ref.** 4, p. 462)

566. (C) The decussating chiasmal fibers involved come from the nasal half of the retinae. In contrast to optic nerve lesions, the vast majority of chiasmal lesions are compressive. (**Ref.** 5, p. 39)

567. (A) This defect, if the progressive lesion is untreated, goes on to involve the nasal fields and produces total blindness. Early, an upper temporal defect may be demonstrated, but this may be asymptomatic. (**Ref.** 5, p. 39)

568. (B) This is a characteristic symptom of pituitary tumor. It occurs because the upward pressure of the tumor interferes with the blood supply of the decussating fibers in the chiasm, and those, as noted above, come from the nasal half of the retinae. (**Ref.** 4, p. 38)

569. (D) An early diagnostic step includes skull films to show sella expansion and thinning of its walls. CT has replaced the need for air encephalography, and NMR (MRI) is generally even better. Angiography, however, may still be necessary. (**Ref.** 4, pp. 236, 246)

570. (C) Two other conditions that may simulate Bell's palsy are polio and disseminated sclerosis. Bell's palsy is sometimes attributed to exposure to a draft and may follow an infection of the nasopharynx. In a small proportion of cases it has been proven to be due to herpes zoster virus, but in most cases no cause is found. (**Ref.** 4, p. 67)

571. (D) Upper and lower facial muscles are usually equally affected. Chorda tympani involvement produces loss of taste on the anterior two-thirds of the tongue, and when the facial nerve lesion extends above the point where the stapedius muscle branch is given off, hyperacusis may occur. (**Ref.** 4, p. 67)

572. (E) The muscles are paralyzed to an equal extent for voluntary, emotional, and associated movements. Displacement of the mouth causes deviation of the tongue to the sound side on protrusion and may cause paralysis of the tongue to be erroneously suspected. (**Ref.** 4, p. 67)

573. (D) Most patients have nearly complete recovery; in a few cases, this may take several months. Permanent severe paralysis is rare. Sometimes the "crocodile tears" phenomenon occurs. (**Ref.** 4, pp. 68–69)

574. (A) Isolated paralysis of one lateral rectus usually means that the lesions involve the nerve at one point between the pons and the orbit. (**Ref.** 4, p. 54)

575. (B) Separation of the images increases the further the eyes are moved in the normal direction of pull of the paralyzed muscle. The false image is displaced in the direction of the planes or planes of action of the paralyzed muscle. (**Ref.** 4, p. 56)

576. (C) The eye is deviated inward by the unantagonized medial rectus. When lateral rectus paralysis is due to a sixth nerve nuclear lesion within the pons, almost invariably one finds associated signs of lesions of other neighboring pontine structures, especially the seventh nerve. (**Ref.** 4, p. 54)

577. (E) Images of a single object formed by the two eyes no longer fall upon the corresponding retinal points. In testing for the false image, colored glasses may be used or each eye may be covered separately. (**Ref.** 4, p. 56)

578. (C) Though possible, craniostenosis deformities more commonly become manifest in the first few years of life rather than this early. In hydrocephalus, enlargement occurs in all diameters. (**Ref.** 5, pp. 485–486)

579. (A) Usually, marked dilatation of the ventricular system is found. CT has now replaced pneumoencephalography. NMR (MRI) gives even more information. (**Ref. 4, pp. 270–271**)

580. (E) The disorder may become arrested. In certain instances, steroids or surgery are helpful. If hydrocephalus is due to an obstruction to the circulation of the CSF at some point, either remove the obstruction, if possible, or bypass it. (**Ref. 4, p. 271**)

581. (E) CT scan is diagnostic in some cases. NMR (MRI), as noted, provides even more data and is helpful in follow-up, whether medical or surgical treatment is employed. (**Ref. 4, pp. 271–272**)

582. (A) Claw hand is commonly found because the extensors are not paralyzed. The triceps reflex is affected. (**Ref. 4, p. 405; Ref. 5, pp. 433–435**)

583. (B) Horner's syndrome results when the lesion is close to the vertebral foramina and involves the sympathetic rami (ie, if the communicating branch to the inferior cervical ganglion is injured). (**Ref. 5, pp. 433–435**)

584. (E) In Klumpke-Dejerine or lower arm paralysis, the eighth cervical and first thoracic roots are injured. Lower radicular syndromes may also be caused by injury to the lower primary trunks. (**Ref. 5, p. 434**)

585. (D) In an affected dermatome or spinal segmental area, there may be hyperesthesia and hyperalgesia or anesthesia and analgesia. Besides the skin, certain deeper structures, namely, bone, joints, and muscles, are also innervated. (**Ref. 4, p. 118**)

586. (C) This is protrusion of the brain; when it contains a cavity communicating with the cerebral ventricles, some refer to it as "hydroencephalocele." If the sac had contained meninges alone, it would have been called a "meningocele"; if only meninges and CSF had been in the sac, the prognosis would have been better. (**Ref. 5, pp. 478–479**)

587. (A) They are found either in the frontal or the occipital regions, often associated with other developmental anomalies. Besides the latter, if large amounts of cerebral tissue are present, if the ventricular system expands into the mass, or if the hydrocephalus is present, the prognosis is worse. (Ref. 5, pp. 478–479)

588. (B) There is a predilection for the muscles of the eyes, face, lips, tongue, throat, and neck. This is caused by a defect of neuromuscular transmission due to antibodies to the acetylcholine receptor; its fluctuating weakness is improved by inhibition of cholinesterase. (Ref. 5, pp. 697–699)

589. (C) The overt pathology is found primarily in the thymus gland. (Ref. 5, pp. 698–699)

590. (E) There is no reaction of degeneration. Single-fiber EMG shows increased jitter and blocking. (Ref. 5, p. 700)

591. (B) The virus appears to be the same as that which causes varicella. Herpes zoster, or shingles, results from the reactivation of the latent virus in a patient who has had chickenpox at some time. (Ref. 4, p. 402)

592. (D) It may complicate any latent virus lesion or the posterior roots. Symptomatic herpes zoster may be precipitated by disturbed autoimmune mechanisms, including those due to immunosuppressive drugs. (Ref. 4, p. 402)

593. (B) Most patients recover without residua, but sometimes intractable pain persists for years in the elderly. One attack usually confers permanent immunity, but second attacks sometimes occur. (Ref. 4, p. 403)

594. (D) Muscular wasting occasionally occurs; encephalitis is rare. The association of pain with sensory loss is occasionally described as "anesthesia dolorosa." (Ref. 4, p. 403)

595. (A) Minimal downward (and inward) movement is effected by the intact fourth cranial nerve. There is also ptosis of the eyelid. (Ref. 5, pp. 418–419)

596. (B) This is found in hemorrhage, ischemia, infarction, and aneurysm. The third nerve is rarely injured by increased intracranial pressure. (**Ref.** 5, pp. 418–419)

597. (B) This is Weber's syndrome; lesions here involve the paramedian aspect of the right side of the mid-brain. Another classic mesencephalic syndrome (Benedikt syndrome) is manifested by crossed hemiataxia and chorea; some include contralateral hemianesthesia. (**Ref.** 5, pp. 212–213)

598. (D) Multiple causes of this kind of lesion include several kinds of hemorrhage, tumor, and aneurysm. CT and NMR (MRI) have been helpful. However, for certain types of lesions (eg, most aneurysms), angiography is still necessary. (**Ref.** 5, pp. 193–203, 418–419)

14

Integrated Chapter

DIRECTIONS (Questions 599–601): Each of the questions or incomplete statements below is followed by five suggested answers or completions. Select the ONE lettered answer or completion that is BEST in each case.

---

599. A 48-year-old woman complained of severe headache and dizziness. Her magnetic resonance angiogram (Figs. 14.1A and 14.1B) was

   A. abnormal, indicating brainstem vascular insufficiency

   B. abnormal, indicating inadequate flow via the right vertebral artery

   C. normal

   D. normal except for moderate asymmetry in caliber of the two A1 segments

   E. abnormal, revealing bilateral intracavernous carotid aneurysms

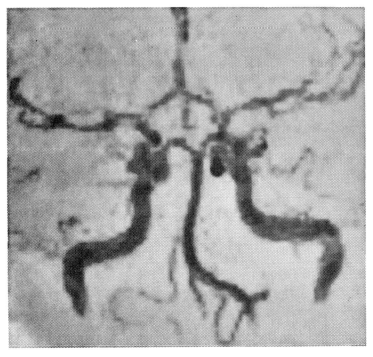

Figure 14.1A.

600. Magnetic resonance angiography (MRA)
   A. is generally able to show aneurysms as small as 2 mm
   B. is particularly helpful in showing early draining veins
   C. is usually valuable in demonstrating neovascularity or blush
   D. routinely visualizes slow flow lesions especially well with entirely non-invasive technique
   E. has demonstrated aneurysms, vascular malformations, and occlusions

601. Arnold-Chiari malformation has been divided into two types such that
   A. in the adult form, surgical enlargement of the foramen magnum and decompression of the cervico-medullary junction is recommended for virtually every case
   B. in the adult form, upbeat nystagmus is characteristic

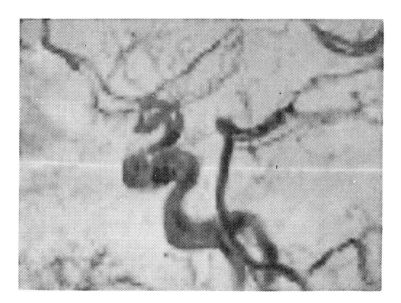

Figure 14.1B.

  C. in the adult form, MRI cannot generally establish the diagnosis unless there are co-existing bony abnormalities

  D. in the infantile form, there has usually been hydrocephalus
in the early months of life

  E. in the infantile form, prognosis is good despite the presence
of extensive defects

DIRECTIONS (Questions 602–606): The group of questions below
consists of lettered headings followed by a list of numbered words or
statements. For each numbered word or statement, select the ONE lettered heading that is most closely associated with it. Each lettered
heading may be selected once, more than once, or not at all.

  A. Lacunar state
  B. Pure sensory stroke
  C. Pure motor hemiplegia
  D. Dysarthria-clumsy hand
  E. Ataxic hemiparesis

---

602. Internal capsule, basis pontis

603. Thalamus

604. Diffuse deep white matter

605. Anterior limb of internal capsule (rarely basis pontis)

606. Basis pontis, cortico-spinal, and cerebellar peduncle tracts

---

DIRECTIONS (Question 607): The incomplete statement below is followed by suggested completions. Select the ONE that is BEST.

---

607. Arousal in fear with poor recall
  A. suggests depression insomnia
  B. occurs at regular intervals throughout sleep
  C. occurs at NREM, first half of night
  D. occurs at REM, second half of night
  E. occurs at the same time of night as does arousal in fear with good recall

---

DIRECTIONS (Questions 608–612): Each group of questions below consists of lettered headings followed by a list of numbered words or statements. For each numbered word or statement, select the ONE lettered heading that is most closely associated with it. Each lettered heading may be selected once, more than once, or not at all.
  A. Hyperactive, dilated pupils, tremor, hyperthermia; blood test diagnostic
  B. Naloxone, 0.4 mg intravenously or intramuscularly; repeat if needed
  C. Agitated, confused, visual hallucinations, dilated pupils, flushed and dry skin
  D. Confused, perceptional distortions, accidents or violence; if severe, panic
  E. Similar to A (above) but less paranoid, more euphoric; blood and urine tests diagnostic

---

608. Phencyclidine (PCP, angel dust)

609. Cocaine

610. Transderm delirium

611. Methylphenidate

612. Methadone, oxycodone

DIRECTIONS (Questions 613–614): Each of the questions or incomplete statements below is followed by five suggested answers or completions. Select the ONE that is BEST in each case.

---

613. In acute head injury, following the immediate or primary brain injury, a secondary brain injury may result from
   A. combination of arterial hypoxemia and arterial hypertension
   B. toxic, breakdown products of blood and abnormal metabolites such as arachidonic acid
   C. complete metabolism of glucose with accumulation of lactic acid in brain and CSF
   D. vasospasm, followed by severe drop in intracranial pressure with subsequent herniation
   E. direct tissue injury under this site of impact, producing, for example, homonymous hemianopsia, even in patients who remain alert

614. A recent large study on antihypertensive treatment for isolated systolic hypertension in the elderly (Systolic Hypertension in the Elderly Program [SHEP] Pilot Study)
   A. showed that elderly people did not tolerate the medication as well as younger people
   B. resulted in a significantly increased incidence of stroke due to decreased perfusion pressure
   C. demonstrated that diuretics must not routinely be used because of their adverse effects on carbohydrate metabolism and angina pectoris
   D. resulted in a significantly decreased incidence of stroke except for patients age 80 or over
   E. resulted in a significantly decreased incidence in stroke for all age groups including patients age 80 or over

DIRECTIONS (Questions 615–619): Each group of questions below consists of lettered headings followed by a list of numbered words or statements. For each numbered word or statement, select the ONE lettered heading that is most closely associated with it. Each lettered heading may be selected once, more than once, or not at all.

    A. Creutzfeldt-Jakob disease
    B. AIDS dementia complex
    C. Subacute sclerosing panencephalitis
    D. Progressive multifocal leukoencephalopathy
    E. Visna, Scrapie

615. Measles virus; myxovirus (RNA)

616. Spongiform encephalopathic agents

617. JC virus; papovavirus (DNA)

618. Retrovirus (RNA) (Lentivirus)

619. Sheep

DIRECTIONS (Question 620): The incomplete statement below is followed by five suggested completions. Select the ONE that is BEST.

620. In Gilles de la Tourette's syndrome
    A. the tics worsen with age
    B. vocal and motor tics, by their nature, are more disabling to the patient than is associated obsessive-compulsive disorder
    C. obsessive-compulsive disorder occurs in more than 90% of the cases
    D. haloperidol, clonazepam, clonodine, and fluoxetine have all been used in treatment
    E. males and females are approximately equally affected

DIRECTIONS (Questions 621–627): Each group of questions below consists of lettered headings followed by a list of numbered words or statements. For each numbered word or statement, select the ONE lettered heading that is most closely associated with it. Each lettered heading may be selected once, more than once, or not at all.

Questions 621–624:

A. Lower motor neuron changes in arms and spasticity in legs, with arms weaker than legs; urinary retention, incontinence; variable sensory involvement with pain and temperature typically reduced in hands

B. Voluntary motor function lost; pain and temperature sensation lost; proprioception and vibratory sensation intact

C. Proprioception and vibratory sensation lost; pain and temperature sensation intact

D. Ipsilateral motor weakness; loss of ipsilateral proprioception and vibratory sensation; loss of contralateral pain and temperature sensation

621. Anterior cord syndrome

622. Central cord syndrome

623. Brown-Sequard syndrome

624. Posterior cord syndrome

Questions 625–627:

A. Respiratory muscle paralysis

B. Some biceps function but weak arm extension, wrist extension

C. Intrinsic hand function weakness but wrist extension retained

625. C8 cord lesion

626. C6 cord lesion

627. Lesion above C4 cord level

DIRECTIONS (Question 628): The incomplete statement below is followed by five suggested completions. Select the ONE that is BEST.

---

628. A highly malignant primary, non-endocrinopathic brain tumor which is very cellular with hyperchromatic nuclei and which seeds the meninges via the CSF is
- **A.** ependymoma
- **B.** medulloblastoma
- **C.** glioblastoma multiforme
- **D.** anaplastic astrocytoma

DIRECTIONS: Each group of questions below consists of lettered headings followed by a list of numbered words or statements. For each numbered word or statement, select the ONE lettered heading that is most closely associated with it. Each lettered heading may be selected once, more than once, or not at all.

Questions 629–633: Vertebro-basilar ischemia has been suggested as a cause of all of the following symptoms and each symptom has an anatomic correlate:

- **A.** Dysphagia
- **B.** Amnestic episodes, transient global amnesia
- **C.** Episodic unconsciousness, drowsy state
- **D.** Visual hallucinations
- **E.** Tinnitus and deafness

629. Cochlear nuclei

630. Reticular activating structures of midbrain and rostral connections

631. Tenth nerve nuclei

632. Bilateral temporal lobe

633. Parietal—occipital region

DIRECTIONS (Question 634): The incomplete statement below is followed by five suggested completions. Select the ONE that is BEST.

---

634. Toxic neuropathy due to
   A. uremia may be accompanied by "burning foot" or "restless leg" syndrome
   B. uremia involves a specific type of proximal axonopathy
   C. uremia is essentially unchanged by successful renal transplantation
   D. uremia is most effectively reversed by chronic hemodialysis
   E. diphtheria and buckthorn are demyelinating conditions which represent two of the many biologic toxins consistently associated with neuropathy

---

DIRECTIONS (Questions 635–639): Each group of questions below consists of lettered headings followed by a list of numbered words or statements. For each numbered word or statement, select the ONE lettered heading that is most closely associated with it. Each lettered heading may be selected once, more than once, or not at all.

   A. Diagnosis of brain death; also used frequently in distinguishing between organic and psychogenic causes of unresponsiveness
   B. Lateral lemniscus
   C. Posterior columns
   D. Suspected meningo-encephalitis
   E. P100 latency prolongation with increased intracranial pressure

635. Lumbar puncture

636. EEG

637. Visual evoked potentials

638. Brainstem auditory evoked potentials

639. Somatosensory evoked potentials

DIRECTIONS (Question 640): The incomplete statement below is followed by five suggested completions. Select the ONE that is BEST.

---

640. In patients with acquired immunodeficiency syndrome
- **A.** approximately one-third have overt neurologic symptoms and/or signs
- **B.** almost all, with or without clinical neurologic manifestations, have HIV detectable in the CSF
- **C.** approximately 10% have central nervous system neuropathologic findings at autopsy
- **D.** HIV has been isolated from brain tissue and cerebrospinal fluid but, due to a membrane barrier, not from spinal cord
- **E.** Zidovudine (formerly Azidothymidine) has been shown to decrease mortality in AIDS but, unfortunately, not to reverse HIV-associated neurologic symptoms and signs

---

DIRECTIONS (Questions 641–645): Each group of questions below consists of lettered headings followed by a list of numbered words or statements. For each numbered word or statement, select the ONE lettered heading that is most closely associated with it. Each lettered heading may be selected once, more than once, or not at all.
- **A.** Infantile form and adult form
- **B.** Associated with sacral hypertrichosis
- **C.** Often associated with neck pain
- **D.** Alone, does not cause neck pain or other neurologic symptoms
- **E.** usually asymptomatic but considered to be a potential cause of back pain

---

641. Klippel-Feil syndrome

642. Facet tropism

643. Diastematomyelia

644. Congenital stenosis of cervical spinal canal

645. Arnold-Chiari syndrome

DIRECTIONS (Question 646): The incomplete statement below is followed by five suggested completions. Select the ONE that is BEST.

---

646. In the differential diagnosis of dementia
  A. CT must be done because, for example, if atrophy is demonstrated, certain patterns are diagnostic of Alzheimer's disease
  B. the possibility of endocrinopathy must be investigated
  C. history of head trauma (specifically recent), meningo-encephalitis or subarachnoid hemorrhage must be sought
  D. any depression, if present, unfortunately will be irreversible
  E. it is important to note that "benign forgetfulness" all too often goes on to become Alzheimer's or Pick's disease

---

DIRECTIONS (Questions 647–661): Each group of questions below consists of lettered headings followed by a list of numbered words or statements. For each numbered word or statement, select the ONE lettered heading that is most closely associated with it. Each lettered heading may be selected once, more than once, or not at all.

Questions 647–651:

  A. Encephalopathy with metabolic alkalosis
  B. Encephalopathy with metabolic acidosis
  C. Encephalopathy with respiratory alkalosis
  D. Encephalopathy with mixed acid-base disorder
  E. Encephalopathy with respiratory acidosis

647. Corticosteroid excess

648. Hypercarbic-anoxic encephalopathy

649. Sepsis; salicylism (adult)

650. Poisoning with salicylates in children; methanol; severe convulsions

651. Pulmonary infiltration; upper brainstem disease

Questions 652–656:

    A. Destroys cranial nuclei and nerves, motor and sensory pathways and cerebellar connections
    B. Germinomas; precocious puberty in boys
    C. Early interference with CSF circulation, causing hydrocephalus
    D. Symptoms and signs of cerebral dysfunction plus cranial nerve, spinal cord, and nerve root involvement
    E. Loss of vestibular response to caloric stimulation; high CSF protein

652. Meningeal carcinomatosis

653. Brainstem glioma

654. Cerebellopontine angle tumor

655. Fourth ventricle tumor

656. Pineal tumors

Questions 657–661:

    A. Loud snoring and obstructed breathing
    B. Coordinated mobility but unresponsive
    C. Uncoordinated mobility but unresponsive
    D. Quiet cessation of breathing
    E. REM's with frightening dreams

657. Narcolepsy

658. Primary sleep apnea

659. Secondary sleep apnea

660. REM sleep without atonia

661. Somnambulism

DIRECTIONS (Question 662): The incomplete statement below is followed by five suggested completions. Select the ONE that is BEST.

---

662. In myelin disorders
  A. peripheral nervous system disease involves oligodendrocytes, central nervous system disease involves Schwann cells
  B. the oligodendrocyte process wraps around a segment of an axon in a concentric fashion to form myelin
  C. vitamin B_{12} deficiency affects peripheral myelin but not central myelin
  D. the leukodystrophies affect central myelin but not peripheral myelin
  E. multiple sclerosis is diagnosed as "clinically definite" if there are two attacks plus clinical evidence of one lesion or one attack plus clinical evidence of two or more lesions

---

DIRECTIONS (Questions 663–671): Each group of questions below consists of lettered headings followed by a list of numbered words or statements. For each numbered word or statement, select the ONE lettered heading that is most closely associated with it. Each lettered heading may be selected once, more than once, or not at all.

Questions 663–667:

  A. Acute brain contusion during first 48 hours
  B. Feeding and draining vessels of AVM
  C. Small intradural masses (eg, neurofibromas and meningeal carcinomatosis)
  D. Metastatic bone disease of spine
  E. Posterior fossa tumors

663. Plain films and radionuclide scan as primary imaging choice

664. MRI

665. CT

666. Arteriography

667. Myelography

Questions 668–671:

  A. Sporadic; main feature is autonomic insufficiency; also, parkinsonism, cerebellar ataxia, dysphagia, laryngeal stridor, amyotrophy
  B. Autosomal dominant; main feature is cerebellar ataxia; also, ophthalmoplegia, parkinsonism, dystonia, optic atrophy, retinal degeneration, amyotrophy, dysphagia, dementia
  C. Sporadic; main features are ptosis and ophthalmoplegia; also, short stature, heart block, cerebellar ataxia, deafness, retinal degeneration, myopathy, Babinski signs, mental deficiency
  D. Sporadic; main feature is ophthalmoplegia, especially vertical; also, gait ataxia, axial dystonia, parkinsonism, pseudobulbar palsy, dementia

  668. Kearns-Sayre syndrome

  669. Progressive supranuclear palsy

  670. Shy-Drager syndrome

  671. Hereditary ataxia, adult type

DIRECTIONS (Question 672): The incomplete statement below is followed by five suggested completions. Select the ONE that is BEST.

---

672. In convulsive disorders
   A. most investigators believe that the fundamental abnormality in all such conditions lies in the cerebral cortex, including the limbic cortex (hippocampus)
   B. in chronic epilepsy, the physiologic abnormality and the recurrent neuronal paroxysms are intermittent
   C. neurons in cortical areas adjacent to the epileptic focus may demonstrate paroxysmal hyperpolarization only, which appears to facilitate epileptic spread during the interictal state
   D. cortico-reticular epilepsy begins on one side of the cortex
   E. seizures stop as a result of neuronal exhaustion

DIRECTIONS (Questions 673–696): Each group of questions below consists of lettered headings followed by a list of numbered words or statements. For each numbered word or statement, select the ONE lettered heading that is most closely associated with it. Each lettered heading may be selected once, more than once, or not at all.

Questions 673–677:

   A. Nutritional demyelinating disorder with severe hyponatremia
   B. Leukodystrophy, in the dysmyelinating disease group
   C. Non-leukodystrophy dysmyelinating disease
   D. Nutritional demyelinating disorder involving corpus callosum and other areas
   E. Viral demyelinating disease

673. Central pontine myelinolysis

674. Pelizaeus-Merzbacher disease

675. Marchiafava-Bignami disease

676. Phenylketonuria

677. Progressive multifocal leukoencephalopathy

Questions 678–682:

    A. Partial and generalized convulsive seizures
    B. Absence
    C. Absence and myoclonus
    D. Partial and absence
    E. All

678. Ethosuximide

679. Clonazepan

680. Carbamazepine

681. Methsuximide

682. Valproic acid

Questions 683–687:

    A. Neurologic sequelae frequently include deafness and seizures
    B. Botulinum toxin
    C. Lisuride, selegiline
    D. Amyloid B-protein and its precursor
    E. Increase of 100% to 200% of amino acid levels in CSF has been reported

683. Parkinson's disease

684. Alzheimer's disease

685. Blepharospasm, spasmodic torticollis, hemifacial spasm

686. Bacterial meningitis

687. Amyotrophic lateral sclerosis

Questions 688–691:

A. Human fetal cell transplants being tried increasingly
B. Lessening optimism regarding adrenal medullary transplants to brain
C. One recent study found antecedent stressful events twice as common in test group compared with control group
D. Various causes suggested include toxins, poliomyelitis virus, metabolic derangement, and genetics defects; current interest in possible role of excitatory amino acids
E. Ongoing trials of infusion of nerve growth factor into ventricles of patients with this disorder

688. Stroke

689. Parkinson's disease

690. Alzheimer's disease

691. Amyotrophic lateral sclerosis

Questions 692–696:

A. Most can communicate by vertical eye movements
B. Schizophrenia or severe depression
C. Spontaneous unarousability interruptable only by vigorous, direct external stimulation
D. Sustained, complete loss of self-aware cognition with autonomic functions relatively intact
E. Often associated with factitious responses to stimulation

692. Stupor

693. Locked-in state

694. Catatonic state

695. Hysteria-malingering

696. Vegetative state

DIRECTIONS (Questions 697–700): Each of the questions or incomplete statements below is followed by suggested answers or completions. Select the ONE that is BEST in each case.

---

697. In restless legs syndrome
  - **A.** the neurologic examination occasionally reveals hyperactive reflexes in the lower extremities
  - **B.** the movements begin during REM sleep
  - **C.** like akathisia, sleep is disrupted
  - **D.** clonazepan or levodopa have been beneficial
  - **E.** no correlation with iron deficiency anemia has been found but the syndrome has been associated with pregnancy, rheumatoid arthritis, and uremia

698. The first report of the North American Symptomatic Carotid Endarterectomy Trial indicated that in
  - **A.** symptomatic patients with severe (70% to 99%) stenosis, endarterectomy reduced stroke risk 17%
  - **B.** asymptomatic patients with severe (70% to 99%) stenosis, endarterectomy reduced stroke risk 17%
  - **C.** asymptomatic patients with moderate (30% to 69%) stenosis, endarterectomy reduced stroke risk 17%
  - **D.** symptomatic patients with moderate (30% to 69%) stenosis, endarterectomy reduced stroke risk 17%
  - **E.** symptomatic patients with severe (30% to 99%) stenosis, endarterectomy reduced stroke risk 17%

699. In post-traumatic stress disorder
  - **A.** it is almost impossible to differentiate this from generalized anxiety disorder
  - **B.** the major treatment is neuropharmacological
  - **C.** affected persons are drawn to activities that evoke recollection of the traumatic event
  - **D.** patients often exhibit a "hyper-emotional" responsiveness or involvement with the world after the trauma

    E. symptoms include hyperalertness, "startle response," sleep disturbance, guilt, and difficulties with memory and concentration

700. In serious electrical injury to the nervous system
    A. electric shock therapy is the most common cause
    B. late manifestations of electrical injury are common
    C. basal ganglia injury is the most frequent late manifestation
    D. CNS lesions are most likely due to direct effect of the current
    E. atrophic paralysis is the most frequent late manifestation

Answers and Discussion

599. (C) Asymmetry of the vertebral arteries is a fairly frequent occurrence and alone does not indicate pathology. Sometimes the larger vertebral artery is called "dominant." The smaller vertebral artery might represent a potential source of focal, inadequate collateral circulation in the presence of additional stress factors (eg, decreased perfusion secondary to shock). (**Ref.** 9, pp. 84, 2058; **Ref.** 20, pp. 1369–1376)

600. (E) MRA, a non-invasive procedure, has been able to demonstrate aneurysms, vascular malformations and occlusions; aneurysms as small as 4 (sometimes 3) mm have been shown by this technique. Certain physiologic information such as arteriovenous circulation time, early draining veins, and neovascularity or blush is lacking. Slow flow lesions can sometimes be visualized if additional measures (eg, gadolinium injection) are used. Newer modifications of MRA are expected to solve these problems in the very near future. (**Ref.** 9, pp. 84, 2058; **Ref.** 20, pp. 1369–1376)

601. (D) In the infantile form, surgical therapy is attempted via ventricular shunting for the hydrocephalus and repair of the meningomyelocele. Prognosis is poor for patients with extensive defects. In the adult form, MRI establishes the diagnosis even when there are no coexisting bony abnormalities. In the adult form, downbeat nystagmus is characteristic. Surgical therapy in the adult form requires careful selection of cases. (**Ref.** 9, p. 2258)

2

602. (C)   This is one of the more common types of lacunar strokes. It disrupts the corticospinal tracts. (**Ref. 9**, p. 2167; **Ref. 5**, p. 215)

603. (B)   This involves the sensory nucleus of the thalamus. (**Ref. 9**, p. 2167; **Ref. 5**, p. 215)

604. (A)   In lacunar strokes, the individual lesions are less than 3 mm in diameter but they may be multiple and occasionally coalesce to form larger areas visible by CT. (**Ref. 9**, p. 2167; **Ref. 5**, p. 215)

605. (D)   This is a less common variety of lacunar stroke. (**Ref. 9**, p. 2167; **Ref. 5**, p. 215)

606. (E)   This type also involves the posterior limb of the internal capsule. (**Ref. 9**, p. 2167; **Ref. 5**, p. 215)

607. (C)   This suggests night terrors and nightmares. In REM sleep, subjects are easily aroused and often report detailed and vivid dreams. Depression insomnia is associated with frequent postural shifts during the second half of the night. (**Ref. 9**, p. 2078)

608. (D)   Milder symptoms and signs include: wide-eyed, dilated pupils; restless, hyperreflexia; less often, hypertension or tachycardia. (**Ref. 9**, p. 2069)

609. (E)   Severe symptoms and signs include: arrhythmia, occasional convulsions. (**Ref. 9**, p. 2069)

610. (C)   Severe symptoms and signs include: florid, toxic disoriented delirium; later, amnesia, fever; hot, flushed dry skin. (**Ref. 9**, p. 2069)

611. (A)   Severe symptoms and signs include: assaultive; occasional convulsions, hypothermia, circulatory collapse. (**Ref. 9**, p. 2069)

612. (B)   Severe symptoms and signs include: coma; pinpoint pupils, hypotension, hypothermia. (**Ref. 9**, p. 2069)

613. (B)   Arachidonic acid metabolism may release oxygen-free radicals in the production of prostaglandins. Glucose may be metabolized incompletely. Arterial hypotension may be present. Intracranial pressure may elevate. (**Ref.** 9, p. 2239)

614. **(E)** This (SHEP) study was the first to identify a treatment benefit for any form of hypertension in patients 80 years of age or older. (**Ref.** 21, pp. 3255, 3301)

615. **(C)** This involves defective viral gene expression. (**Ref.** 9, p. 2203)

616. **(A)** Relatively rapid dementia and myoclonus in adult patient with normal CSF. (**Ref.** 9, pp. 2203, 2206)

617. **(D)** Insidious onset, steady progression; begins focally but proceeds to multifocal, bilateral abnormalities. (**Ref.** 9, pp. 2203, 2207)

618. **(B)** This is a primary neurologic disorder also referred to as subacute encephalitis (or encephalopathy) or AIDS encephalopathy. (**Ref.** 9, p. 2203)

619. **(E)** Visna is caused by a retrovirus and somewhat resembles HIV infection of the nervous system. Scrapie resembles Creutzfeldt-Jakob disease and Kuru. (**Ref.** 9, p. 2203)

620. **(D)** A recent study using Fluoxetine, an antidepressant that inhibits serotonin uptake, has reportedly shown improvement in both Tourette's syndrome and obsessive-compulsive disorder. Haloperidol unfortunately affects personality ("zombie" effect) and school performance; in addition, the patient may develop tardive dyskinesia later. Males are more often affected. The tics become less severe with age. (**Ref.** 9, pp. 2151–2152; **Ref.** 22, pp. 872–874)

621. **(B)** Anterior and lateral columns of cord are dysfunctional; posterior columns intact. (**Ref.** 9, p. 2245)

622. **(A)** Motor fibers to the legs lie more peripherally. Urinary retention-incontinence often present. (**Ref.** 9, p. 2245)

623. **(D)** Dysfunction of half of the cord. (**Ref.** 9, p. 2245)

624. (C) Clinical picture is opposite that of anterior cord syndrome and the prognosis of posterior cord syndrome is better. (**Ref.** 9, p. 2245)

625. (C) Therefore, splints applied to wrist and fingers will give fingers pincer function. (**Ref.** 9, p. 2245)

626. (B) Also, impairment of finger flexion. (**Ref.** 9, p. 2245)

627. (A) Many patients die. (**Ref.** 9, p. 2245)

628. (B) Metastatic tumors may also seed CSF (meningeal carcinomatosis). Pineal tumors may produce endocrinopathy and seed CSF. Although medulloblastomas are radiosensitive, long-term follow-up may show radiation damage. (**Ref.** 9, pp. 2230, 2234, 2235)

629. (E) A less common symptom of vertebro-basilar ischemia and origin doubtful if the two symptoms occur alone. (**Ref.** 9, p. 2169)

630. (C) The central reticular formation is the anatomical basis of an alerting system. (**Ref.** 4, pp. 168–169; **Ref.** 9, p. 2169)

631. (A) Unilateral damage to the nucleus ambiguus usually produces only slight dysphagia, but bilateral damage causes aphagia. (**Ref.** 5, pp. 427–428)

632. (B) When this was first described, recurrence had not been noted; later on, recurrence was found (though rarely). (**Ref.** 9, p. 2169)

633. (D) Binocular visual loss is much more frequent a symptom of vertebro-basilar ischemia. (**Ref.** 9, p. 2169)

634. (A) The axonal change is non-specific. Uremic polyneuropathy is prevented and reversed by successful renal transplantation but chronic hemodialysis is often ineffective in reversing it. (**Ref.** 9, pp. 2265–2266)

635. (D) Because of the development of brain imaging, lumbar puncture is performed much less than before. However, it is still indispensable in diagnosing several infectious diseases and is an emergency procedure in cases of suspected bacterial meningitis. **(Ref. 9, p. 2056)**

636. (A) Absence of EEG activity supports the diagnosis of brain death. **(Ref. 9, p. 2056)**

637. (E) This may also be elevated in degenerative neurologic disorders. P100 latency is related to conduction in the optic nerve and central visual pathways. **(Ref. 9, p. 2056)**

638. (B) The first potential recorded is generated by the auditory nerve. **(Ref. 9, p. 2056)**

639. (C) Median or peroneal nerves are most often stimulated. **(Ref. 9, p. 2056)**

640. (A) 30% to 40% of HIV-infected patients with no evidence of neurologic abnormalities have HIV detectable in the CSF. As many as 90% of patients with AIDS have CNS neuropathologic findings at autopsy, including the spinal cord. **(Ref. 23, pp. 695–699)**

641. (D) However, when associated with coexisting anomalies of the CNS (eg, syringomyelia), neurologic symptoms and signs are found. **(Ref. 9, p. 2257)**

642. (E) Some believe that facet misalignment increases rotational stress on the facet joints and causes back pain. **(Ref. 9, p. 2257)**

643. (B) This bony abnormality divides the spinal canal leading to duplication of the spinal cord. **(Ref. 9, p. 2258)**

644. (C) When this occurs in the lumbar region, back pain and neurologic disability can occur. **(Ref. 9, p. 2258)**

645. (A) Infantile form is often associated with other midline defects and the presence of extensive defects yields a poor prognosis. In the adult form, certain carefully selected cases may benefit from surgical treatment. (**Ref.** 9, p. 2258)

646. (B) Hypothyroidism and other treatable disorders (eg, vitamin B_{12} deficiency), must not be overlooked. Depression may present as pseudodementia and can be reversed with treatment of the depression. Benign forgetfulness does not in itself lead to dementia. Cerebral atrophy demonstrated by CT or MRI can be consistent with, but not diagnostic of, Alzheimer's disease. (**Ref.** 9, p. 28)

647. (A) Severe chloride or potassium depletion can produce this. (**Ref.** 9, p. 2067)

648. (E) Pulmonary insufficiency, central or peripheral ventilatory paralysis also causes this. (**Ref.** 9, p. 2067)

649. (D) Fulminant hepatic encephalopathy can be the basis. (**Ref.** 9, p. 2067)

650. (B) Uremia or diabetic ketoacidosis are also causative. (**Ref.** 9, p. 2067)

651. (C) Hepatic encephalopathy may also produce this picture. (**Ref.** 9, p. 2067)

652. (D) Carcinoma, sarcoma, lymphoma, leukemia, and glioma. (**Ref.** 9, p. 2231)

653. (A) Cranial nerve palsies, weakness, sensory disturbance, ataxia, and nystagmus. (**Ref.** 9, p. 2231)

654. (E) Acoustic schwannoma: tinnitus, hearing loss, nystagmus, vertigo; brain stem signs. (**Ref.** 9, p. 2231)

655. (C) Ependymoma, medulloblastoma: hydrocephalus, vomiting, brainstem/cerebellar signs. (**Ref.** 9, p. 2231)

656. (B) Neurologic: hydrocephalus, paralysis of upward gaze. (**Ref.** 9, p. 2231)

657. (E) These tend to occur at the onset of sleep. (**Ref.** 9, p. 2078)

658. (D) This occurs during deep sleep or initiating sleep. (**Ref. 9,** p. 2078)

659. (A) This occurs repeatedly throughout sleep. (**Ref.** 9, p. 2078)

660. (C) This is observed from REM sleep; patients may injure themselves or their bed partners. (**Ref.** 9, pp. 2078–2079)

661. (B) This is observed from NREM sleep; stairways, gates, or other physical restraints may help. (**Ref.** 9, pp. 2078–2079)

662. (B) Central myelin is an extension of the oligodendrocyte, which manufactures the myelin sheath. Vitamin B_{12} deficiency and also the leukodystrophies affect both central myelin and peripheral myelin. CNS disease involves oligodendrocytes; peripheral nervous system disease involves Schwann cells. A diagnosis of "clinically definite" multiple sclerosis requires two attacks plus clinical evidence of two lesions with other conditions ruled out. (**Ref.** 9, pp. 2211, 2213, 2259)

663. (D) MRI subsequently is indicated because of greater sensitivity in detecting intraosseous metastases. (**Ref.** 9, p. 2060)

664. (E) MRI is superior to CT for both intra-axial and extra-axial tumors here because of absence of bone-induced artifacts, better resolutions, and relatively high contrast between normal and abnormal tissues. (**Ref.** 9, p. 2060)

665. (A) Later on, MRI is superior for small hemorrhages. (**Ref.** 9, p. 2060)

666. (B) Arteriography also is best for showing the precise anatomy of an aneurysm. (**Ref.** 9, p. 2060)

667. (C) However, in meningeal carcinomatosis, even myelography may remain normal in more than half of the cases. (**Ref.** 9, p. 2060)

668. (C) Cerebellar ataxia, deafness, retinal degeneration, myopathy, Babinski signs, mental deficiency. (**Ref.** 9, p. 2153)

669. (D) Parkinsonism, pseudobulbar palsy, dementia. **(Ref. 9, p. 2153)**

670. (A) Dysphagia, laryngeal stridor, amyotrophy. **(Ref. 9, p. 2153)**

671. (B) Dystonia, optic atrophy, retinal degeneration, amyotrophy, dysphagia, dementia. **(Ref. 9, p. 2153)**

672. (A) In chronic epilepsy, although the seizures themselves are intermittent, the physiologic abnormality persists throughout the interictal period. Neurons in cortical areas adjacent to the epileptic focus may demonstrate paroxysmal hyperpolarization only, forming an *inhibitory surround* that appears to prevent epileptic spread during the interictal state. Corticoreticular epilepsy concerns generalized seizures, and these begin bilaterally. Seizures stop because of neuronal exhaustion plus self-activating inhibitory mechanisms. **(Ref. 9, pp. 2217–2218)**

673. (A) Occurs one to three days after a period of profound hyponatremia followed by rapid osmolal correction of greater than 20 mEq per liter. **(Ref. 9, pp. 2140, 2211)**

674. (B) Affects males only, sex-linked recessive, starts in early infancy, progresses slowly throughout cerebrum and cerebellum; peripheral nervous system not affected. **(Ref. 9, pp. 2211, 2216)**

675. (D) Rare, affects middle-aged men who are severely addicted to various kinds of alcoholic beverages; progressive dementia, recovery rate. **(Ref. 9, pp. 2140, 2211)**

676. (C) Normal at birth but if unrecognized, child develops, during first year of life, mental retardation, tremors, seizures, eczema, hypopigmentation, and hyperactivity. **(Ref. 9, p. 1155)**

677. (E) Progressive deterioration in mental status and the evolution of focal neurologic deficits in absence of meningismus or CSF abnormalities. Serial CT's diagnostic of this demyelinating disorder. **(Ref. 9, p. 2211)**

678. (B) Still the drug of choice for absence seizures because it is safer than valproic acid. **(Ref. 9, pp. 2226–2227)**

679. (C) May lose effectiveness with time as tolerance develops. (**Ref.** 9, pp. 2226–2227)

680. (A) May be preferred over phenytoin because of latter's disturbing cosmetic side effects. (**Ref.** 9, pp. 2226–2227)

681. (D) Can be used alone or as adjunctive medication. (**Ref.** 9, pp. 2226–2227)

682. (E) Can produce serious hepatic side effects that laboratory tests may not predict. (**Ref.** 9, pp. 2226–2227)

683. (C) Combination of selegiline and low dose levodopa appears to be an effective initial treatment. (**Ref.** 24, p. 3134)

684. (D) The macromolecule is found in cells and blood vessels in the brains of patients with Alzheimer's disease. (**Ref.** 24, p. 3135)

685. (B) Injections of botulinum toxin have been useful; the toxin is a potent blocker of the neuromuscular junction and has few of the side effects of other blockers. (**Ref.** 24, p. 3135)

686. (A) No longer the scourge it once was, its neurologic sequelae still include brain damage. (**Ref.** 24, p. 3135)

687. (E) If excitatory amino acids do, in fact, play a role, newer therapies are possible. (**Ref.** 24, p. 3134)

688. (C) The stroke did not immediately follow the stressful experience and therefore some kind of prevention might be feasible. (**Ref.** 24, p. 3135)

689. (A, B) More long-term follow-ups of adrenal medullary transplant patients show less impressive results whereas fetal cell transplants may be more effective and retain viability longer. (**Ref.** 24, p. 3134)

690. (E) In experimental animals, these infusions preserve neurons whose axons have been severed. (**Ref.** 24, p. 3135)

691. (D) One such excitatory amino acid (ie, glutamate) damages neurons exposed to high levels of this neurotransmitter. (**Ref.** 24, p. 3134)

692. (C) Coma refers to a state of unarousable unresponsiveness; even strong stimuli don't elicit recognizable psychological responses. (**Ref.** 9, p. 2061)

693. (A) This is a pseudocoma, that is, a state resembling acute unconsciousness but with self-awareness preserved. (**Ref.** 9, p. 2061)

694. (B) An uncommon type of pseudocoma which resembles organic stupor. No pathologic reflexes are found and all neurologic laboratory tests (eg, imaging studies, EEG, etc.) are normal. (**Ref.** 9, p. 2061)

695. (E) A pseudocoma with unarousable unresponsiveness, usually brief and unaccompanied by physiologic abnormalities. (**Ref.** 9, p. 2061)

696. (D) Wake/sleep cycles are intact, for example. (**Ref.** 9, p. 2061)

697. (D) Therefore, some investigators believe that the syndrome results from an underactive dopaminergic system. The neurologic examination, however, is normal, the movements most often occur during light, non-REM sleep. Akathisia rarely disrupts sleep. It has been associated with iron deficiency anemia as well as the other conditions named in (E). (**Ref.** 25, p. 3014)

698. (A) This is the only subset of patients who reportedly benefitted from the surgical treatment. The first report was not able to find benefit for asymptomatic patients or those with 30% to 69% stenosis. (**Ref.** 26, pp. 711–720)

699. (E) In these disorders, there is the presence of a clear antecedent that is recognizable as potentially causing symptoms of distress in almost anyone; this differentiates it from generalized anxiety disorder. The major treatment is psychotherapeutic, especially group sessions, although medications may be useful (eg, if panic or depression are also present). The patients avoid activities that could evoke recollection of the traumatic event and they often show a lack of emotional responsiveness or involvement with the world after the trauma. (**Ref.** 9, p. 2101)

700. (**E**)   This is a result of injury to the peripheral nerves or spinal cord. The most common cause of electrical injury is accidental contact with high-tension currents in the home or industry. Late manifestations are rare. Hemiplegia and other focal cerebral symptoms, chorea, dystonia, and other signs of basal ganglia injury have been reported. CNS lesions are more probably due to damage to blood vessels or to cerebral anoxemia secondary to the temporary cardiac and respiratory failure. (**Ref.** 5, p. 445)

References

1. Slosberg P. Chapter VIII—Non-operative management of ruptured intracranial aneurysms. *Clin Neurosurg.* 1974;21:90–99. (Williams &Wilkins, Baltimore) 1974.

2. Slosberg P. Zero per cent mortality due to recurrent hemorrhage in follow-up of medically treated ruptured single intracranial aneurysms: a 23-year study. *Trans Am Neurol Assoc.* 1979;104:180–183.

3. Huckman MS. Normal pressure hydrocephalus: evaluation of diagnostic and prognostic tests. *AJNR.* 1981;2:385–395.

4. Brain L. *Clinical Neurology.* 6th ed. London: Oxford University Press; 1985.

5. Rowland LP. *Merritt's Textbook of Neurology.* 8th ed. Philadelphia: Lea & Febiger; 1989.

6. Gastaut H. Clinical and electroencephalographical classification of epileptic seizures. *Epilepsia.* 1970;11:102–119.

7. Slosberg P. Symptomatic unruptured giant aneurysms: medical treatment. *Acta Neurochir.* 1982;62:207–208.

8. Lusins J, Nakagawa H, Bender MB. Unoperated bilateral subdural hematoma. *NY State J Med.* 1980;80:1869–1871.

9. Wyngaarden JB, Smith LH. *Cecil Textbook of Medicine.* 18th ed. Philadelphia: W.B. Saunders; 1988.

10. Post KD, Flamm ES, Goodgold A, Ransohoff J. Ruptured intracranial aneurysms; case morbidity and mortality. *J Neurosurg.* 1977;46:290–295.

11. Slosberg P. Senior citizen with ruptured aneurysm: in Viewpoint (with Drake CG). *Neurosurgery.* 1980;6:605–606.

12. Slosberg P. Treatment and prevention of stroke: Part II. *NY State J Med.* 1973;73:758–763.

13. Gross JA, Haas ML, Swift TR. Ethylene oxide neurotoxicity: report of 4 cases and review of the literature. *Neurology.* 1979; 29:978–983.

14. Bruno J, Wilder BJ. Valproic acid. Review of a new epileptic drug. *Arch Neurol.* 1979;36:393–398.

15. Aring C. A medical perspective. *Neurology.* 1984;34:1357–1361.

16. Krieger HP. Therapy for cranial aneurysm (Letter). *Arch Neurol.* 1986;43:7–8.

17. Hashimoto N, Kang Y, Yamazoe N, Nakatani H, Kikuchi H, Hazama F. Experimental study on the pathogenesis and non-surgical treatment of saccular cerebral aneurysms. *Stroke Supplement I.* August 1990;21:I-154, I-155. Abstract.

18. Slosberg P. Very long-term follow-up of patients with ruptured intracranial aneurysms treated entirely medically including 5 patients followed up 30 years or more. *Stroke Supplement I.* August 1990;21:I-145. Abstract.

19. Rinne JO, Roytta M, Paljarvi L, Rummukainen J, Rinne UK. Selegiline (deprenyl) treatment and death of nigral neurons in Parkinson's disease. *Neurology.* 1991;41:859–861.

20. Ross JS, Masaryk TJ, Modic MT, Harik SI, Wiznitzer M, Selman WR. Magnetic resonance angiography of the extracranial carotid

arteries and intracranial vessels: a review. *Neurology.* 1989;39: 1369–1376.

21. SHEP Cooperative Research Group, Prevention of stroke by anti-hypertensive drug treatment in older persons with isolated systolic hypertension. *JAMA.* 1991;265:3255–3264.

22. Como PG, Kurlan R. An open-label trial of fluoxetine for obsessive-compulsive disorder in Gilles de la Tourette's syndrome. *Neurology.* 1991;41:872–874.

23. Tartaglione TA, Collier AC, Coombs RW, et al. Acquired immunodeficiency syndrome. Cerebrospinal fluid findings in patients before and during long-term oral Zidovudine therapy. *Arch Neurol.* 1991;48:695–699.

24 Joynt RJ. Neurology (Contempo '91). *JAMA.* 1991;265:3134–3135.

25. McGee S. Restless legs syndrome (Questions and Answers). *JAMA.* 1991;265:3014.

26. NASCET Steering Committee. North American Symptomatic Carotid Endarterectomy Trial. *Stroke.* 1991;22:711–720.

27. Rolak LA. Literary neurologic syndromes—Alice in Wonderland. *Arch Neurol.* 1991;48:649–651.

28. Nichols D. Endovascular treatment of the acutely ruptured intracranial aneurysm. *J. Neurosurg.* 1993; 79:1–2.

Errata

Slosberg
Medical Examination Review
Neurology
Tenth Edition

Enclosed are replacements for pages
147, 148, 151, 156, 158, 159, 160

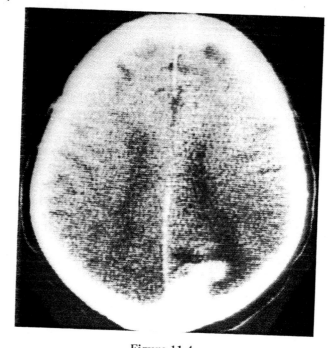

Figure 11.4.

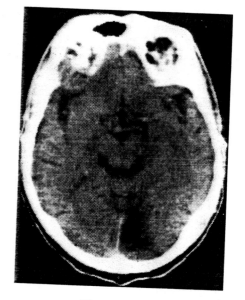

Figure 11.5A.

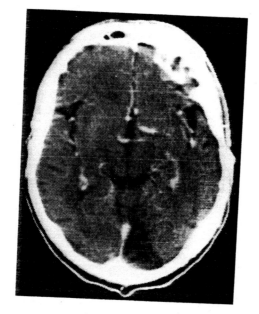

Figure 11.5B.

391. The accompanying angiogram (Fig. 11.6) illustrates a condition
in which

    A. clipping of the neck is almost invariably performed
    B. early surgical treatment produces uniformly good results
    C. late surgical treatment produces uniformly good results
    D. no medical treatment has been reported to be helpful
    E. none of the above

392. The patient whose angiogram is shown (Fig. 11.7) had a subarachnoid hemorrhage. He

    A. has a posterior communicating artery aneurysm
    B. has a middle cerebral artery aneurysm
    C. has an anterior communicating artery aneurysm
    D. will die after a few weeks of recurrent hemorrhage unless
microsurgical treatment is attempted

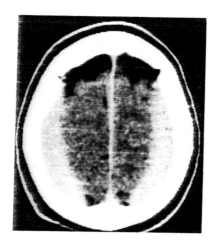

Figures 11.8A. and 11.8B.

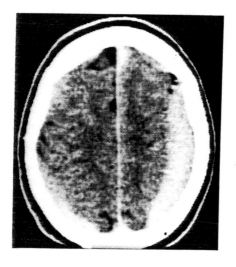

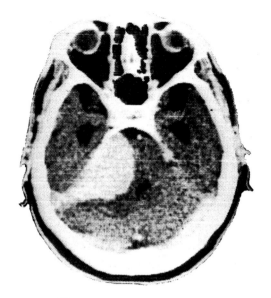

Figures 11.11A. and 11.11B.

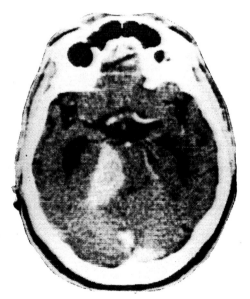

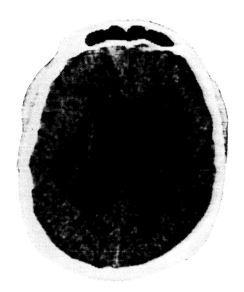

Figure 11.12.

15. In this condition
    A. radionuclide cisternography is generally accepted as the most accurate predictor of shunt success
    B. a callosal angle of less than 90 degrees on CT has been found to have prognostic value regarding surgery
    C. the presence of large lateral ventricles without visualization of the temporal horn tips indicates that the patient is a candidate for surgery
    D. metrizamide CT cisternography has shown promise as an additional predictor of shunt success
    E. clinical improvement after lumbar puncture has no predictive value regarding shunt success

16. In the condition illustrated by the accompanying figures (Figs. 11.13A and 11.13B)
    A. shunting appears to be indicated, at least from a radiographic standpoint

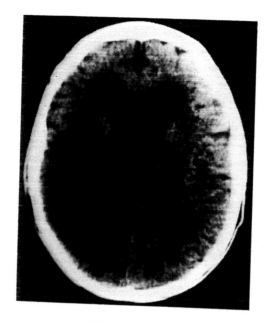

Figure 11.13A.

B. tricyclic treatment often helps
C. in a 41-year-old female this CT would be considered within normal limits
D. Pick's disease is not the first diagnostic choice
E. this plus one other laboratory test together can distinguish Alzheimer's disease from Pick's disease

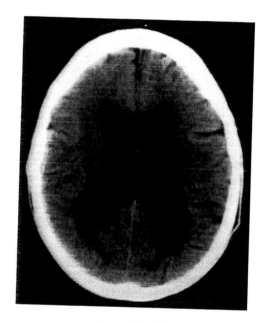

Figure 11.13B.